MEDICAL AND SURGICAL EDUCATION - PAST, PRESENT AND FUTURE

Edited by **Georgios Tsoulfas**

Medical and Surgical Education - Past, Present and Future
http://dx.doi.org/10.5772/intechopen.68660
Edited by Georgios Tsoulfas

Contributors

Anusuiya Subramaniam, Murali Sambasivan, Abu Daud Silong, Lindsay Bank, Mariëlle Jippes, Albert J.J.A Scherpbier, Fedde Scheele, John Weigelt, Travis Webb, Phillip Redlich, Jaime Villalba-Caloca, Javier Pineda-Gutiérrez, Sergio Martínez-Fonseca, Marcelino Alonso-Gómez, Avelina Sotres-Vega, Panteleimon Pantelidis, Angeliki Chorti, Ioanna Papagiouvanni, Georgios Paparoidamis, Georgios Lales, Thrasyvoulos Panagiotakopoulos, Christos Drosos, Michail Sideris, Hadi Mohammadi, Sander Alken, Jan-Maarten Luursema, Cornelia Fluit, Harry Van Goor

Published by InTech
Janeza Trdine 9, 51000 Rijeka, Croatia

Publishing Process Manager Marina Dusevic
Technical Editor SPi Global
Cover InTech Design team

First published March, 2018
Printed in Croatia
Legal deposit, Croatia: National and University Library in Zagreb

Additional hard copies can be obtained from orders@intechopen.com

Medical and Surgical Education - Past, Present and Future, Edited by Georgios Tsoulfas
p. cm.
Print ISBN 978-953-51-3941-6
Online ISBN 978-953-51-3942-3

For EU product safety concerns:
IN TECH d.o.o., Prolaz Marije Krucifikse Kozulić 3, 51000 Rijeka, Croatia,
info@intechopen.com or visit our website at intechopen.com.

Meet the editor

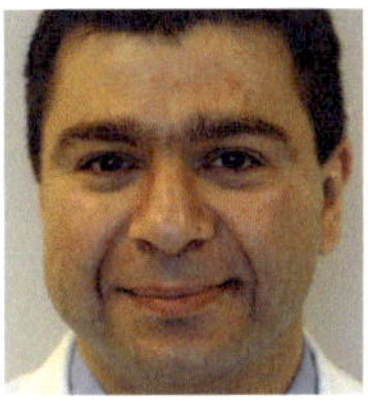

Dr. Georgios Tsoulfas received his medical degree from Brown University School of Medicine and completed his general surgery residency at the University of Iowa Hospitals and Clinics, as well as a transplant research fellowship at the Starzl Transplant Institute at the University of Pittsburgh. He then completed a 2-year transplantation surgery fellowship at the Massachusetts General Hospital, Harvard Medical School, and then joined the Division of Solid Organ Transplantation and Hepatobiliary Surgery at the University of Rochester Medical Center as an Assistant Professor of Surgery. He has currently moved back to Greece, where he is an Associate Professor of Surgery at the Aristoteleion University of Thessaloniki. He has published over 70 papers in peer-reviewed journals and in PubMed, as well as 17 book chapters. He is a reviewer of 15 international journals and is on the Editorial Board of several others.
He is currently the Vice-Chair of the International Relations Committee of the American College of Surgeons and the World President of the International College of Surgeons.

Contents

Preface

The last century has witnessed tremendous changes in the education and training system of medical students, as well as medical and surgical residents, in short, our future physicians. This has been the result of changes in the educational philosophy, the technology, and the needs of our patients, just to name a few. We have learned that medical and surgical education is not simply about providing medical knowledge, but finding out a way to impart this knowledge together with the love for medicine in such a way that they will inspire young physicians, as well as prepare them for the difficult task ahead.

A key challenge is to learn more about the various systems in medical education throughout the world and identify advantages and disadvantages, a process from which we can all (and most importantly our patients) benefit from. This book is a compilation of the experiences, thoughts, and "best-practice" advice of a panel of international experts on medical and surgical education. It also offers us a glimpse of the immediate future with chapters discussing the implementation of new technology in medical education (such as augmented and virtual reality), as well as better management strategies with the use of block time.

Georgios Tsoulfas, MD, PhD, FICS, FACS
Associate Professor of Surgery
Aristotle University of Thessaloniki
Thessaloniki, Greece

Chapter 1

Integrating Technical and Nontechnical Skills in Hands-On Surgical Training

Alexander PB Alken, Cornelia Fluit,
Jan-Maarten Luursema and Harry van Goor

Additional information is available at the end of the chapter

http://dx.doi.org/10.5772/intechopen.73044

Abstract

Safe and effective surgery requires high-quality technical and nontechnical skills. Although the importance of nontechnical skills has become increasingly clear, today's surgical curricula still lack formal training in nontechnical skills. In this chapter, we discuss how to integrate technical and nontechnical skills training into surgical curricula and provide strategies on how to teach both skill sets concurrently in a hands-on setting.

Keywords: surgical training and teaching, operating room teaching, technical skills, nontechnical skills, communication and team skills, integrated technical and nontechnical skills training, concurrent technical and nontechnical skills training

1. Introduction

The operating room is a hectic and dynamic teamwork environment requiring safe surgical practice. To achieve this, surgeons have to develop highly effective technical and nontechnical skills that are both built upon formal training [1]. Since technical and nontechnical skills are strongly associated to another [1] and have to be applied concurrently in the real-life operating room, these skills also have to be trained concurrently [2–5]. However, to date, the training of nontechnical skills is still not effectively and fully implemented in surgical curricula [1].

Surgical curricula have always had a strong focus on the development of surgical technical skills, aiming for high-level psychomotor skills, swift eye-hand coordination, and dexterity [6]. Since it became clear that adverse events in surgery are not so much caused by deficiencies and errors in technical skills but rather by deficiencies and errors in nontechnical team and communication skills, the attention for nontechnical skills training has been increasing [1, 7].

In this chapter, we discuss how to effectively integrate technical and nontechnical skills in surgical curricula, focusing on teaching behaviors, training strategies, and simulated and real-life operating room training. We address the current knowledge on acquiring technical skills in the section "How do we learn and teach surgical technical skills?" and nontechnical skills in "How do we learn and teach nontechnical skills in surgery?". We discuss training settings used for concurrent technical and nontechnical skills training in "Environments used for teaching nontechnical skills next to technical skills in surgery." We address frameworks that can be helpful to integrate technical and nontechnical skills teaching in the section "Effective frameworks for integrated technical and nontechnical skills teaching." Finally, we share our view on how to successfully establish a surgical curriculum with integrated technical and nontechnical skills training and teaching in "Integrating technical and nontechnical skills training during hands-on surgical teaching in a curriculum".

We realize that nontechnical skills of surgeons encompass more than communication and team skills, such as clinical decision making and stress coping [5]. In this chapter, the term 'nontechnical skills' refers to the social team and communication skills necessary for successful surgery, encompassing effective communication (e.g., sharing information efficiently), collaboration (e.g., assisting other team members when needed), coordination (e.g., timely asking team members for requests), leadership (e.g., directing team members), and situational awareness (e.g., asking for information updates regarding the patient's condition) [8, 9].

2. How do we learn and teach surgical technical skills?

Technical skills are core skills of a surgeon. They refer to all goal-directed psychomotor actions. Handling a scalpel to gain access to a patient's abdomen and handling a needle to repair a ruptured vein are examples of technical surgical skills. We discuss the current knowledge available regarding the learning, training and teaching of technical skills, and surgical technical skills in particular.

To understand how technical skills are acquired, two main principles are important. First, the acquisition of technical skills is not a linear process [10]. At the start of training, trainees are completely unfamiliar and inexperienced. There are many untrained aspects of the skill that can be improved relatively easily resulting in a rapid growth of trainees during their first trials. After the first trials, however, the basics of the skill are acquired and the speed of progress starts to slow down. All aspects of the skill are familiar but now have to be optimized, which requires much more time. The second principle regarding the acquisition of technical skills involves the way a skill is cognitively approached by trainees. In the beginning stages of learning, trainees depend on explicit rules to perform the skill that demands extensive cognitive effort. In later stages, the skill is partially or completely automated and trainees are less dependent on rules. Performing the skill then requires far less cognitive effort and enables trainees to focus on other actions, activities, or aspects in the training or working environment [10]. Both principles are important for designing the training and the teaching that is to be provided.

Distributed, short training sessions with sufficient resting periods in between are most effective to acquire technical skills [10]. Effective training stimulates trainees to engage in deliberate practice, meaning that trainees repetitively train skills in a dedicated and conscious manner according to clear and achievable learning goals. Training of skills has to be simple at the start and complexity should gradually increase over time in accordance to each trainee's individual progress and needs. Teaching has to contain demonstrations, instructions, and immediate feedback intensely in case of novice trainees [10] to prevent the wrong acquisition and automation of skills [11]. But as trainees progress, this intensity should be reduced accordingly and feedback should be increasingly given reflectively [10] (**Figure 1**). Highly frequent feedback stimulates the initial acquirement of skills in the short term, whereas less frequent feedback seems to stimulate the retention of the learned skills in the long term. If tasks enable trainees to derive perceptual feedback and trainees are able to evaluate and improve their skills themselves, no feedback may be required. Under such circumstances intense feedback can even hamper learning [10]. Feedback has to be provided in a constructive manner [12]. Based on first-hand observations, teachers should provide specific information to trainees regarding what went well and what needs to be improved [12]. All teaching has to occur in a calm, supportive, and respectful way to create a safe and effective teaching climate [13, 14]. The use of neutral, nondisturbing language is essential in achieving this [15]. When teaching technical skills, the information density should be limited to how to perform the skill without focusing on other aspects or additive information (e.g., other options and the environment) [11]. Such information can prevent trainees from learning because executing the task and simultaneously processing the teaching require trainees to process too much information, which can easily cause cognitive overload. It is also important that trainees can learn by exploring and committing errors to experience firsthand what works best and what possible consequences are [10]. Simulation training plays an important role here.

2.1. Effective teaching behavior

Research to effective surgical skills teaching is primarily based on trainees', teachers', and educational experts' perceptions of effective teaching. Furthermore, research relating teachers' teaching behaviors to the actual acquisition of trainees' skills is scarce, especially in surgical and other medical training. This makes it hard to determine evidence-based how teachers exactly should teach. A recently conducted systematic review study on technical skills teaching in medicine, sports, and music found that feedback, instructions, suggestions for improvement, and demonstrations by teachers improved the skills development in trainees (Medical

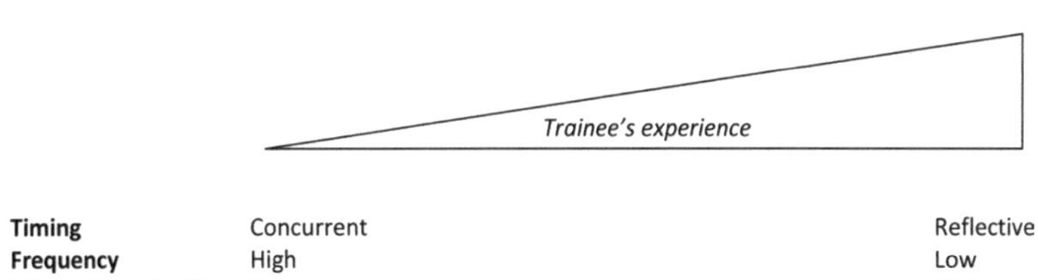

Figure 1. Changes in feedback on technical skills according to the trainee's progress.

Teacher, paper under review [16]). It was also found important that teachers stimulated trainees to verbalize their thoughts and reasoning processes. A safe training environment was also found to be important. However, it remained unclear how these behaviors should exactly look like in order to effectively improve the acquisition of skills in trainees. Only one behavior was found to be sufficiently supported by evidence and was described elaborately: instructions and feedback that made trainees externally focus on the task and the effect was more effective than instructions and feedback that made trainees internally focus on how to exactly move their body parts. It may be more effective to explain by "When suturing, move the needle in a circular motion as if you are going to make a full circle." than by "When suturing, move your wrist with a turning motion.". However, results were only shown in psychomotor sport skills teaching. It is unclear whether it is also effective in surgical hands-on training.

3. How do we learn and teach nontechnical skills in surgery?

Most nontechnical skills trainings are built upon (the combination of) three approaches: theory-based, demonstration-based, and simulation-based training [1]. In the theory-based training, trainees are classroom-like taught what nontechnical skills are, why they are important, and how they can be applied in the operating room. Demonstration-based training adds demonstrations of nontechnical skills to the theory-based approach. Trainees observe, for example, video-recordings of a simulated operation and discuss the behaviors they have seen, possible consequences, and solutions. Both approaches are low cost and easily organized. Both approaches improve trainees' knowledge, awareness, and attitudes. However, there are no possibilities for trainees to apply and train nontechnical skills by doing. Simulation-based approaches do have a training-by-doing component. Trainees apply and train nontechnical skills hands-on in a safe environment, varying from simple bench-top models to full-scale simulated operating rooms with, for example, a patient simulator. This enables the hands-on training of basic and advanced nontechnical skills in a realistic and multidisciplinary team setting. Simulation training is easily compatible with the theory-based and demonstration-based approaches. Simulation has been shown to improve skills acquisition, both in training and in the real-life operating room. Drawbacks are that simulation training is costly, demands extensive organization since realistic operating teams have to be composed, and requires guidance by trained teachers. Blended approaches in which theory, demonstrations, and simulations are combined are advocated. Theory and demonstrations should be the focus in the early stages of nontechnical skills training. In following stages, nontechnical skills should be applied and trained in simulated settings [1, 4]. Simulation has been shown to be most effective in acquiring nontechnical skills [2]. Nontechnical skills training should be long-term, structured according to learning goals, trainees' individual needs and experiences, and firmly embedded into surgical training curricula [1, 4]. Multiple and distributed training sessions are considered most effective [2].

Although simulation training has been shown to be effective within different surgical specialties [2], the applied interventions are often minimally described [17]. As a consequence, it remains unclear how nontechnical skills teaching should exactly look like to be effective [1].

Most commonly used are debriefing sessions immediately after simulation in which reflective feedback on nontechnical skills is provided by a teacher [2]. Debriefing sessions are considered highly important for teaching nontechnical skills. Trainees receive feedback on their nontechnical skills performance, but also reflect on their nontechnical skills [15]. Teacher feedback on nontechnical skills has to be based on first-hand observations of trainees' performance and has to address specific strong points, weaknesses, and suggestions for improvement. It should always be provided in a respectful way and with a neutral tone of voice. Teachers have to structure their feedback based on observations and evaluations according to nontechnical skills assessment tools [1, 15]. Training is essential to enable surgical teachers to effectively analyze and teach nontechnical skills [1, 2, 15]. Extensive training and coaching by nontechnical skills experts are required.

4. Environments used for teaching nontechnical skills next to technical skills in surgery

4.1. The operating room

To date, surgical trainees generally learn nontechnical skills informally and unstructured *as they pass by* in the real-life operating room [1]. Teaching in the operating room is a challenging task in itself since the patient's safety is the most important aspect that often pushes teaching and training to the background [18]. Teaching as it occurs in the operating room is almost entirely focused on technical skills [15]. The same goes for debriefing sessions after the operation [19]. Nontechnical skills teaching remains to be undertaught [15] and surgical teachers are not sufficiently trained to teach nontechnical skills [1]. Nontechnical skills are not yet a part of the surgical educational culture and teachers are inclined to avoid it, often unaware. This means that the real-life operating room is not the best place to teach and train nontechnical skills, especially when trainees lack technical experience.

4.2. Simulation

Simulation offers surgical teachers the possibility to put the teaching of trainees in the forefront [18]. Trainees can train and apply skills and build experience in a safe environment without any risks for patients. For the training of technical skills, synthetic bench top models, box trainers, virtual reality simulators, animal cadavers, human cadavers, and live animal models are commonly used [20, 21]. Recently, nontechnical skills have slowly been added to the skill sets trained by simulation. Possibilities to integrate nontechnical skills next to technical skills training have been developed, for example by using simulated operating rooms with live animal models [22], manikins, and/or synthetic or hybrid models [18].

4.3. Animal model simulation

Using an animal model adds to the reality of the experience in a simulated operating room. Trainees have to deal with real bleedings, time pressure, and hectic teamwork within realistic operating teams [22]. This reality is considered to contribute to the transfer of the acquired nontechnical skills to the real-life operating room [2]. However, our research showed that integrating technical and nontechnical skills during a training using live animal models remained difficult and resulted in a main focus on the teaching of technical skills and hardly on nontechnical skills [22, 23]. It was assumed that the use of a live animal made training activities too unstable to properly teach nontechnical skills next to technical skills. The animal's condition can really deteriorate without being able to pause the situation. Like in the real-life operating room, the main focus may remain on keeping alive the animal patient and on the technical skills necessary to do so. The teaching of nontechnical skills may easily shift to the background. Furthermore, the occurrence of stress caused by real bleedings, for example, is known to cause cognitive overload. This may have further limited the teachers in teaching nontechnical skills [22].

4.4. Simulated human patient operation

A simulated operating room equipped with an operating table, equipment, instruments, and synthetic or virtual reality models offers more opportunities for integrating nontechnical next to technical skills teaching than other environments [20]. The use of synthetic or virtual models creates the possibility to teach and train surgical procedures and the necessary technical skills in an authentic setting. By adding a realistic operating team, the teaching and training of nontechnical skills are possible. Such simulation setting not only offers extensive debriefing possibilities after simulation, for example with the help of video-recordings but also offers the possibility to freeze the condition of the patient in time. Pause and reflect procedures focused on nontechnical skills can then follow immediately, even in acute situations [22]. While still in the simulation, trainees receive feedback and have the opportunity to immediately apply and train the improved nontechnical skills during the remainder of the simulation. However, no research has yet been conducted to the effectiveness of such pause and reflect procedures.

5. Effective frameworks for integrated technical and nontechnical skills teaching

Many frameworks are available for teaching surgical skills and skills in general. We discuss four approaches that in our opinion are superior at the moment in contributing to the effective integration of technical and nontechnical skills teaching in surgery.

5.1. The Peyton four step approach

The Peyton four step approach is a widely accepted method to teach and train technical medical and surgical skills [11] (**Table 1**). During the first step, the teacher shows the trainee how to perform the skill without any instruction. This is to enable the trainee to entirely focus on the performed motor skills without potentially distracting verbal information. During the second step, the teacher shows and explains the skill according to manageable, logically sequenced part-tasks (steps within the skill). Explanations should be limited to only the key information

	Teacher	Trainee
1	Performs	Observes
2	Shows and explains	Observes
3	Performs	Instructs
4	Observes	Explains and performs

Table 1. Peyton four step approach for technical skills.

to prevent cognitive and information overload. In the third step, the teacher performs the part-tasks according to the instructions provided by the trainee. This enables the teacher insight into the trainee's understandings and misunderstandings and helps the teacher to adjust the teaching. During the fourth step, the trainee first verbalizes what to do in each part-task (the teacher checks whether the part-tasks are understood) and then executes the skill (the teacher checks whether the skill is performed correctly). Misunderstandings or mistakes have to be immediately corrected to teach the skill correctly and prevent the wrong automation of the skill. Although widely used, the evidence for the effectiveness of the Peyton four step and similar approaches is limited [11].

5.2. The Zwisch model

The Zwisch model guides teachers in tailoring their teaching and granting autonomy in accordance to each individual trainee's level for each surgical procedure [24]. The model's first stage, 'show and tell,' applies to inexperienced trainees. The teacher performs the procedure, shows, and explains how it is done, while the trainee observes and assists. This step looks similar to the second step of the Peyton approach; however, the Zwisch model does also allow teaching beyond the key information (e.g., background information, other options, and information on team skills) if the trainee's level of experience allows this. When the trainee is familiar with the entire procedure and is able to actively assist (e.g., anticipating on the progress of the procedure), the trainee moves on to the second stage, 'smart help.' In this stage, the teacher switches between self-performing and assisting the trainee in performing the procedure. The trainee performs most of the procedure based on the teacher's continuous instructions and feedback. This stage continues until the teacher deems the trainee able to perform the entire procedure with this 'smart help.' During the third stage, 'dumb help,' the trainee performs the procedure entirely while the teacher assists and only provides feedback and instructions for fine-tuning the trainee's skills. The final step is called "no help" during which the teacher monitors the trainee performing the procedure and only provides minimal advice. The Zwisch model is supported by psychomotor learning theories [24]; however, research on the effectiveness is mostly lacking.

5.3. The BID model

The three-phase briefing-intraoperative teaching-debriefing (BID) framework [25] has been shown to be effective in structuring the teaching before, during, and after hands-on surgical training in the operating room [13, 14]. The briefing phase is characterized by discussing and setting learning goals for trainees to work on during the intraoperative phase [25, 26]. Trainees come up with learning goals or teachers do suggestions, for example, based on their prior experiences with the trainee. Generally, trainees are inclined to focus on technical skills [14] so teachers may have to stimulate trainees to formulate nontechnical learning goals. Research suggests that if clear learning goals on nontechnical skills are lacking the teachers' attention for nontechnical skills will be minimal [22]. The teacher and trainee should agree to focus on one or two learning goals [25], which help the teacher, but also the trainee, to focus on what has to be taught and trained during the intraoperative phase. The briefing generally takes only a few minutes.

The teaching during the intraoperative phase should be aimed at achieving the learning goals and form the guidelines for the teacher to structure the training [25]. How to effectively teach during the intraoperative or the hands-on training phase is discussed in the sections concerning the learning of technical and nontechnical skills.

The final phase is the debriefing during which the teacher and trainee reflect on the achievement of the learning goals [25]. Research showed that teachers during the debriefing are inclined to emphasize what went wrong with a focus on technical skills and without sufficient elaboration on how to improve [14]. A teacher-trainee dialog should be established containing honest and specific strong points, weaknesses, suggestions, and solutions for future practice based on the formulated learning goals. Also the underlying schemes why trainees acted the way they acted during the intraoperative phase should be discussed [25]. This provides both the trainee and the teacher insight into the trainee's thoughts, beliefs, and reasoning processes. This offers reflection and deeper learning for trainees and provides teachers with the opportunity to specifically develop or improve trainees' schemes regarding technical, and in particular nontechnical skills. Along this process, teachers should preferably ask open questions. Debriefing sessions should always result in individual learning goals for trainees' future performance [15]. The use of video-recordings of the trainee's performance has been shown to be effective in debriefing [2]. It helps and teaches trainees to reflect. Mistakes can be discussed and remediated.

5.4. The 4 C/ID model

The 4 component instructional design (4 C/ID) model is specifically designed for the teaching of complex skills [27, 28] (**Figure 2**). The model distinguishes four components for designing a successful training program: learning tasks, supportive information, procedural information, and additional part-task training. The learning tasks are at the core of the 4 C/ID model and encompass the training of whole-task procedures in an authentic and realistic training setting *from the very start*. Whole-task procedures require trainees to combine knowledge, skills, and attitudes and enable them to train these aspects in a realistic relation to each other. This is an important contrast to classical learning theories, which generally prescribe the division of complex tasks into subtasks for training. The 4 C/ID model considers such an approach only effective for the learning of simple skills or skills that can be automated through training. Obviously, confronting a trainee with a new, complex task at

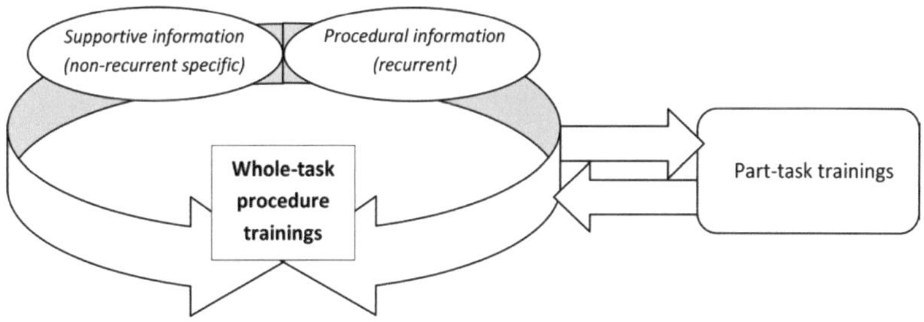

Figure 2. The 4 components of the 4 C/ID-model.

the very start of training will induce cognitive overload and hinder learning. To prevent this, the whole-task training should start with the simplest or most simplified version of this task. This requires much less information processing, reasoning, and problem-solving. As trainees improve, they develop schemes and automate skills that then require less cognitive resources and enable them to focus on other aspects of the skill. As trainees' capabilities improve, the complexity of training should gradually increase accordingly. Whole-task training will improve the effective transfer of the trained skills to real practice, which also requires the whole task to be performed [27, 28]. Regarding the training of technical and nontechnical skills, the 4 C/ID model would require trainees to train these skills concurrently from the very start. Training should gradually progress from the simplest to the most complex version of a surgical procedure.

Supportive information should be available for trainees during training [27, 28]. Supportive information encompasses knowledge that trainees need for reasoning and problem-solving during nonrecurrent, situation-specific aspects of the learning task, for example, information on consequences based on patient-specific characteristics (technical skills) or operating team composition (nontechnical skills). Procedural information encompasses knowledge of recurrent procedural aspects of the learning task [27, 28]. Preferably, this information is provided to trainees during training when the situation requires it, for example, conducting a physical test on the patient (technical skills) or working with a checklist (nontechnical skills) during the operation. Supportive information and procedural information encompass the teaching activities applied by the teacher. The final component of the 4 C/ID model is additional part-task training [27, 28]. Although whole-task training is key and remains the focus during the entire training program, some skills require a high level of automation and additional training. Such skills can be trained and automated in separate training sessions.

The development of and research to integrated technical and nontechnical skills training in surgical specialties are very scarce [5]. Currently, modules are focused on developing technical skills or nontechnical skills, but barely on integrating and developing both skill sets concurrently. Although the 4 C/ID model is built upon solid learning principles and theories, to our knowledge, its effectiveness has not yet been investigated in relation to surgical teaching. Nevertheless, we believe this model helps to integrate technical and nontechnical skills teaching successfully.

6. Integrating technical and nontechnical skills training during hands-on surgical teaching in a curriculum

In this section, we put the aforementioned theory together and share our view on how to effectively integrate technical and nontechnical skills training and teaching in surgical curricula, using both simulated settings and the real-life operating room. We advocate a surgical curriculum to be organized in different training modules. Each training module is composed out of different training sessions. In these training sessions, the actual teaching and training takes place. We provide recommendations on three main aspects: learning goals and assessment; training modules and training sessions; and teaching and training within training sessions.

6.1. Learning goals and assessment

To ensure the formal and structural training of nontechnical skills next to technical skills, long-term learning goals on nontechnical skills have to be formulated next to long-term learning goals on technical skills. Long-term learning goals are formulated by program directors in cooperation with surgical teachers. All have to be achieved by trainees during the curriculum. The long-term learning goals on nontechnical skills can be based on research (for example, the studies conducted by Hull et al. [8] and/or Yule et al. [9]) combined with specific needs of the workplace.

Based on the long-term learning goals, the program directors and surgical teachers formulate short-term learning goals (**Figure 3**). Short-term learning goals have to be achieved by trainees during the training modules within the curriculum. Short-term learning goals address both general and procedure-specific technical and nontechnical skills. General learning goals apply to all surgical procedures. Procedure-specific learning goals specifically apply to distinctive surgical procedures.

The formulated short-term learning goals are the guidelines for the surgical teachers and trainees to formulate personal learning goals for each individual trainee. These personal learning goals enable teachers to tailor the teaching to each individual trainee's needs, experience, and interests. Personal learning goals are specific and achievable. They can be achieved in one or in multiple training sessions.

Each trainee's individual performance and progress is assessed and monitored with assessment instruments on technical skills (like the Objective Structured Assessment of Technical Skills (OSATS)) and nontechnical skills (like the Observational Teamwork Assessment for Surgery (OTAS) [8] or Nontechnical Skills for Surgeons (NOTSS) [9]). The trainees' progress on nontechnical skills is structurally analyzed after each training session and documented with the purpose to provide trainees with feedback and personal learning goals and to improve future performance in upcoming training sessions. Each training module finishes with a summative pass or fail test for trainees on technical and nontechnical skills concurrently, according to the short-term learning goals.

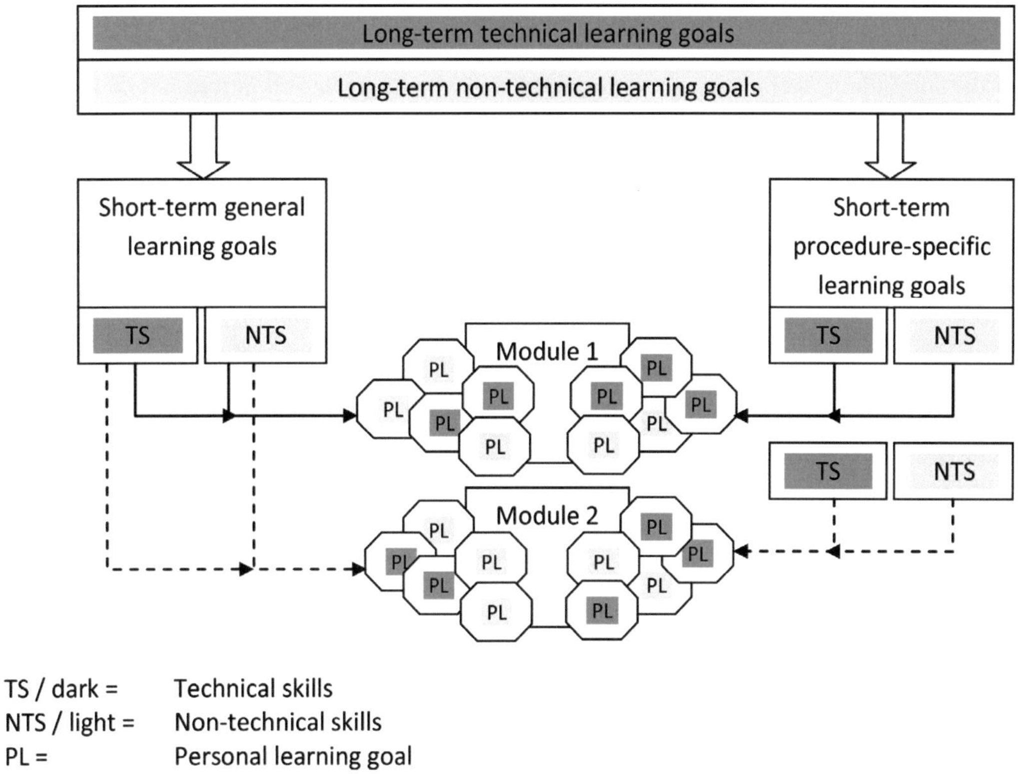

Figure 3. Modular structure of a curriculum for integrated skills' teaching and learning.

Surgical teachers have to be trained and coached in observing, assessing, and teaching nontechnical skills by nontechnical skills teaching experts. Teachers should regularly reflect on their nontechnical and technical skills teaching abilities based on peer observations and feedback. Assessing the teachers' abilities is not a goal in itself but rather a method to strive for perfection, learn from each other, and stay up-to-date regarding effective surgical teaching research and frameworks.

Preferably, nontechnical skills are integrated over the entire line of surgical education, starting in undergraduate medical education all the way through to continuing postgraduate surgical education. It may well be that technical skills require more training and teaching effort to develop than nontechnical skills. The perfect ratio is not known. However, effective nontechnical skills can only be achieved through a formal, structured, and sufficient installation of training possibilities.

6.2. Training modules and sessions

We advocate that surgical training curricula are composed out of training modules focused on specific surgical procedures (e.g., a laparoscopic cholecystectomy module, an open inguinal hernia repair module, etc.). What training modules are exactly incorporated in a curriculum is decided by the program directors depending on the relevance of the modules and the intentions of the curriculum. Technical and nontechnical skills are integrated from the start of a module so trainees learn that both skills are connected and have to be applied and trained concurrently.

6.2.1. Integrated training sessions

A training module consists out of several distributed training sessions. Two types of training sessions are distinguished: integrated training sessions and focused training sessions. Integrated training sessions focus on the teaching and training of both technical and nontechnical skills concurrently within the same training session, in a simulated setting, or in the real-life operating room. If trainees have no prior experience, a training module may typically start with an integrated training session in which trainees purposefully observe and analyze their teachers' technical and nontechnical skills (e.g., based on observational assignments and observational instruments) while their teachers are performing simple versions of the procedure in the real-life operating room. The following integrated training sessions are gradually organized, in accordance to each trainee's individual level, progress, and needs, from:

- *Simple or simplified versions to complex versions of the procedure*

  Gradually moving from simple to complex ensures that trainees do not experience cognitive overload and can start performing procedures or components of procedures themselves in an early stage.

- *Highly controlled simulated to barely controlled real-life training environments*

  Gradually working from a highly controlled to a barely controlled environment ensures there is sufficient room for teaching technical and nontechnical skills, especially in the early stages of training. A highly controlled environment is characterized by simulation, which enables pause and reflect procedures and learning from mistakes. A typical barely controlled environment is the real-life operating room. As trainees start to perform skills themselves, they start in a simple simulation setting (e.g., bench top models). Depending on the trainee's progress, simulated environments become gradually less controllable, increasingly realistic and more and more replaced by training in the real-life operating until the point of independent practice is reached.

- *Teaching of high intensity to teaching of low intensity*

  The teaching intensity gradually fades from strict guidance and intensive teaching in trainees who are inexperienced to distant observation by the teacher with reflective feedback only when trainees are experienced. The Zwisch model can help teachers to determine the necessary teaching intensity.

- *Low trainee contribution to high trainee contribution*

  Trainee contribution gradually increases on the way to independent practice. Trainees first train and apply only the simple components of the procedure, scattered throughout the integrated training sessions. The more complex components are still performed by the teacher. Since full procedure training is important, trainees then purposefully observe and analyze the technical and nontechnical skills still performed by their teacher or assist their teacher during the complex components. As trainees progress, next to the already trained components, increasingly more complex technical and nontechnical components of the procedure are added until trainees can perform the entire and complex versions of the procedure independently. The Zwisch model can be helpful for teachers to gradually grant trainees more autonomy.

6.2.2. *Focused training sessions*

Although the integration of nontechnical next to technical skills training is key, there is also room for focused training. When surgical procedures require skills that need to be automated (e.g., suturing) or require deeper understanding (e.g., models for closed loop communication), supplementary focused training sessions are installed with the specific goal to solely focus on, train, and acquire specific skills. If skills like suturing or closed loop communication are concurrently trained next to other technical and nontechnical skills, it may cause cognitive overload. Then, teaching and training best occurs separately until the skills are partly or fully automated. As soon as these skills are acquired, trainees apply them in the integrated training sessions. By then, trainees are experienced on that part of the procedure and have more cognitive resources available to focus on other important technical and nontechnical skills. Focused training sessions typically occur in a simulated setting, with or without a teacher being present, depending on the possibility for perceptual feedback. With some skills, after the teacher explained the skill by the Peyton four step approach, for example, the trainee can independently practice to automation with at-home training kits, simulators, etc. **Figure 4** provides examples of training in simulated settings, both for focused training (A and B) and integrated training (C).

6.2.3. *Individualized modules*

When applying the aforementioned training and teaching principles, it is important to realize that there is no one size fits all approach. In close and continuous consultation, surgical teachers and trainees individualize each training module and the training sessions within each training module, according to each individual trainee's experience, progress, needs, or interests. Skills and abilities that are already obtained move to the background to enable focus on other skills and abilities. The length of each training module is flexible and different per individual trainee depending on the trainee's speed of progress. Different training modules do not necessarily succeed each other but rather run parallel or partly parallel if similarities in difficulty, techniques, and trainee requirements allow. The basic principle is and remains the training of entire surgical procedures in which both technical and nontechnical skills have to be applied, starting simple and gradually move on to a highly complex endpoint. Along this process, ideally, trainees are guided by two or maximum three teachers within a module; that way, teachers get to know their trainees' strengths and weaknesses, which helps the teacher to tailor the teaching, but also offers trainees feedback from different perspectives.

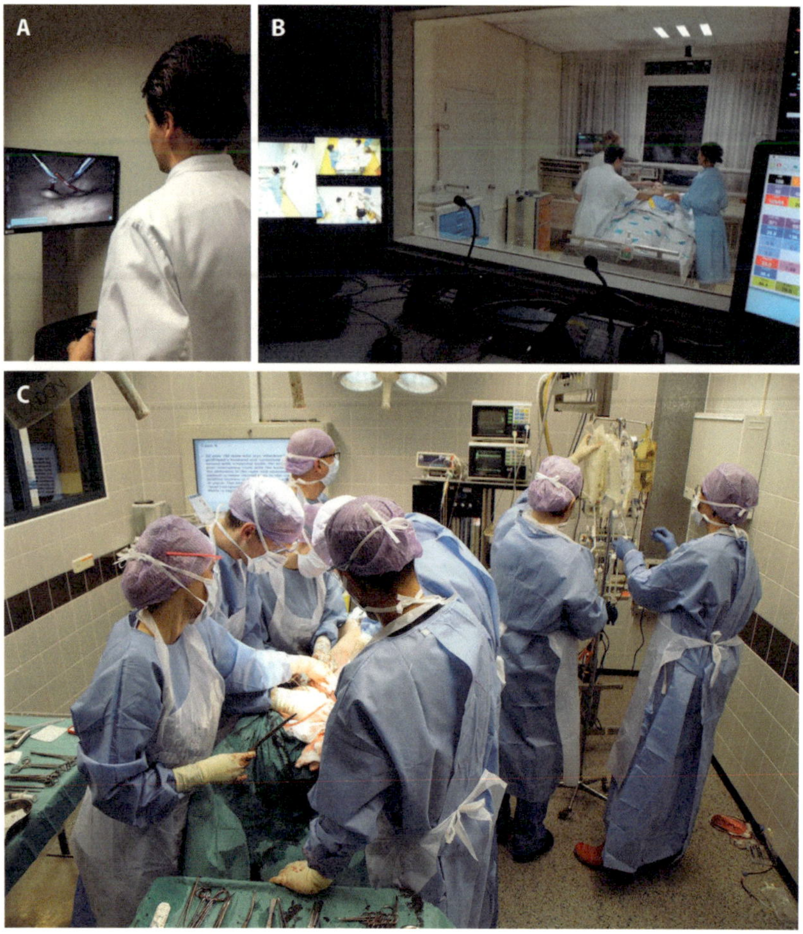

Figure 4. Three simulated training settings, ranked from least realistic and most controlled (A) to most realistic (B) and least controlled (C). (A) A focused training session regarding technical laparoscopic skills using a virtual reality simulator. Basic laparoscopic skills are automated before trainees apply them in the operating room. (B) A focused training session regarding nontechnical communication and team skills using a human patient simulator with video recordings for debriefing (view from control room). Additional training may occur next to training in the real-life operating room. (C) An integrated training session using an animal model. Such training is scheduled best if trainees have gained sufficient experience regarding the necessary technical and nontechnical skills.

6.3. Within training sessions

Good teaching during training sessions is important to develop trainees. Teaching best occurs supportive and in a safe environment. This requires teachers to take time and be calm, approachable, and respectful. Good teaching contains instructions, explanations, demonstrations, and honest feedback with suggestions for improvement tailored to each individual trainee's needs and level. Effective feedback is constructive, nonoffensive, and neutrally formulated. The trainee's strong points and weaknesses are addressed based on and illustrated with first-hand observations. The goal of feedback is to improve or maintain the trainee's level of performance in the future.

The BID model can be helpful to structure the teaching within training sessions. During the briefing, the teacher and trainees briefly discuss and agree on personal learning goals for the upcoming training session, the guidance expectations, and the training activities. Guidance can range from strict and continuously to distant and minimal. Training activities can vary from observing to performing the entire procedure. In integrated training sessions, the teacher and trainee work on one technical and one personal nontechnical learning goal. In focused training sessions, the teacher and trainee work on either one or two technical or one or two nontechnical personal learning goals.

During the hands-on training phase, the actual teaching and training take place. How the teacher teaches depends on the nature of the training session (integrated or focused) and the trainees' experience. Observational learning, a high level of teaching intensity, and a low level of trainee contribution are typical for inexperienced trainees. Distant monitoring, a low level of teaching intensity, and a high level of trainee contribution are typical for experienced trainees. The Zwisch model can help teachers to grant autonomy and determine the teaching intensity.

During technically focused training sessions, trainees are preferably only taught how to perform skills technically (by the Peyton four step approach, for example). Teaching is predominantly directive and instructive and trainees' mistakes are corrected immediately. During nontechnically focused training sessions, teaching may occur more reflective, in debriefings or pause and reflect procedures. If, for example, a communication model is new to trainees, they may first receive short instructions, then observe good and wrong examples, and then immediately apply the skill in a simulated setting. The trainees learn by the feedback provided and reflective questions asked by the teacher. Central questions may be: Why did it go the way it went (addressing both positive and corrective aspects)? Why did you act the way you acted? What are the (possible) consequences? What are the solutions for future practice? Video-recordings of the trainees' performance may be helpful.

In integrated training sessions, teaching focuses on both technical and nontechnical skills concurrently. However, if some technical or nontechnical skills are not yet sufficiently understood or trained, also within integrated training sessions, there can be episodes of pure technical and nontechnical skills teaching. More focused training sessions may be required and can be installed according to the teacher's insight or on the trainee's request.

Each training session closes with a debriefing. A debriefing can typically start with the teacher asking the trainee what he or she thinks went well and needs to be improved, with a special focus on the trainee's personal technical and nontechnical learning goals. The teacher has observed and analyzed the trainee's performance, preferably by using OTAS or NOTSS (nontechnical skills) and OSATS (technical skills). Observations may focus on a few points, adjusted to the trainees' personal learning goals. The teacher provides feedback in a dialog with the trainee and tries to get thoughts, beliefs, and reasoning processes clear. The teacher supports the trainee in his or her development by adding knowledge and expertise to the discussion. The briefing finishes with the trainee formulating future personal learning goals or intentions for the next training.

Author details

Alexander PB Alken[1]*, Cornelia Fluit[2], Jan-Maarten Luursema[1] and Harry van Goor[1]

*Address all correspondence to: sander.alken@radboudumc.nl

1 Department of Surgery, Radboud University Medical Center, Nijmegen, The Netherlands

2 Health Academy, Radboud University Medical Center, Nijmegen, The Netherlands

References

[1] Hull L, Sevdalis N. Advances in teaching and assessing nontechnical skills. Surgical Clinics. 2015;**95**(4):869-884

[2] Dedy NJ et al. Teaching nontechnical skills in surgical residency: A systematic review of current approaches and outcomes. Surgery. 2013;**154**(5):1000-1008

[3] Dawe S et al. Systematic review of skills transfer after surgical simulation-based training. British Journal of Surgery. 2014;**101**(9):1063-1076

[4] Whittaker G et al. Teamwork assessment tools in modern surgical practice: A systematic review. Surgery Research and Practice. 2015:1-11. Article ID 494827

[5] Brunckhorst O et al. The relationship between technical and nontechnical skills within a simulation-based ureteroscopy training environment. Journal of Surgical Education. 2015;**72**(5):1039-1044

[6] Agha RA, Fowler AJ, Sevdalis N. The role of non-technical skills in surgery. Annals of Medicine and Surgery. 2015;**4**(4):422-427

[7] Gjeraa K et al. Non-technical skills in minimally invasive surgery teams: A systematic review. Surgical Endoscopy. 2016;**30**(12):5185-5199

[8] Hull L et al. Observational teamwork assessment for surgery: Content validation and tool refinement. Journal of the American College of Surgeons. 2011;**212**(2):234-243.e5

[9] Yule S et al. Surgeons' non-technical skills in the operating room: Reliability testing of the NOTSS behavior rating system. World Journal of Surgery. 2008;**32**(4):548-556

[10] White C, Rodger MW, Tang T. Current understanding of learning psychomotor skills and the impact on teaching laparoscopic surgical skills. The Obstetrician & Gynaecologist. 2016;**18**(1):53-63

[11] Nicholls D et al. Teaching psychomotor skills in the twenty-first century: Revisiting and reviewing instructional approaches through the lens of contemporary literature. Medical Teacher. 2016;**38**(10):1056-1063

[12] LeBlanc VR et al. 18 Simulation in Postgraduate Medical Education. Members of the FMEC PG consortium. 2011:1-26

[13] McKendy KM et al. Perioperative feedback in surgical training: A systematic review. American Journal of Surgery. 2017;**214**(1):117-126

[14] Timberlake MD et al. What do we know about intraoperative teaching?: A systematic review. Annals of Surgery. 2017;**266**(2):251-259

[15] Spanager L et al. Comprehensive feedback on trainee surgeons' non-technical skills. International Journal of Medical Education. 2015;**6**:4

[16] Alken A et al. Teaching complex surgical psychomotor skills in the OR: A systematic review. Journal of Surgical Education. Submitted

[17] Gordon M, Darbyshire D, Baker P. Non-technical skills training to enhance patient safety: A systematic review. Medical Education. 2012;**46**(11):1042-1054

[18] Kneebone R et al. Distributed simulation—Accessible immersive training. Medical Teacher. 2010;**32**(1):65-70

[19] Ahmed M et al. Actual vs perceived performance debriefing in surgery: Practice far from perfect. The American Journal of Surgery. 2013;**205**(4):434-440

[20] Palter VN, Grantcharov TP. Simulation in surgical education. Canadian Medical Association Journal. 2010;**182**(11):1191-1196

[21] Sadideen H et al. Simulators and the simulation environment: Getting the balance right in simulation-based surgical education. International Journal of Surgery. 2012;**10**(9):458-462

[22] Alken A et al. Integrating technical and non-technical skills coaching in an acute trauma surgery team training: Is it too much? The American Journal of Surgery. 2017. In press

[23] Alken A et al. Feedback activities of instructors during a trauma surgery course. The American Journal of Surgery. 2013;**206**(4):599-604

[24] DaRosa DA et al. A theory-based model for teaching and assessing residents in the operating room. Journal of Surgical Education. 2013;**70**(1):24-30

[25] Roberts NK et al. The briefing, intraoperative teaching, debriefing model for teaching in the operating room. Journal of the American College of Surgeons. 2009;**208**(2):299-303

[26] Meyerson SL et al. Defining the autonomy gap: When expectations do not meet reality in the operating room. Journal of Surgical Education. **71**(6):e64-e72

[27] Van Merriënboer JJ, Kirschner PA, Kester L. Taking the load off a learner's mind: Instructional design for complex learning. Educational Psychologist. 2003;**38**(1):5-13

[28] Janssen-Noordman AM et al. Design of integrated practice for learning professional competences. Medical Teacher. 2006;**28**(5):447-452

Chapter 2

The Indirect Effects of Participative and Abusive Supervisions on Talent Development through Clinical Learning Environment

Anusuiya Subramaniam, Murali Sambasivan and
Abu Daud Silong

Additional information is available at the end of the chapter

http://dx.doi.org/10.5772/intechopen.72119

Abstract

This chapter aims to examine the indirect effect of clinical learning environment in the relationship between supervisory styles (participative and abusive supervisions) and talent development in the healthcare setting. A questionnaire-based survey was implemented to collect the data. The data was collected from 355 junior doctors in six Malaysian public hospitals. The partial least squares based structural equation modeling (PLS-SEM) was used to test the hypotheses. The main findings are: (1) clinical learning environment has a strong positive indirect effect on the participative supervision-talent development link. This reveals that a conducive clinical learning environment that allows empowerment leads to talent development and (2) clinical learning environment has a strong negative indirect effect on the abusive supervision-talent development link. This implies that junior doctors who feel abused have reduced capacity to work and participate in the learning environment which consequently affects their talent development. The result of this study is consistent with theoretical propositions that clinical learning environment indirectly affects the relationship between participative supervision-talent development and abusive supervision-talent development. This study contributes to the clinical learning environment literature by providing empirical support towards identifying clinical learning environment as the underlying mechanism that accounts for the participative supervision-talent development and abusive supervision-talent development relationships.

Keywords: participative supervision, abusive supervision, clinical learning environment, talent development, public hospitals

INTECH
open science | open minds

1. Introduction

Human capital is an organization's greatest asset. Attracting and retaining the right talents are critical to the success of an organization. An organizations' main priority is in human resource development (HRD) to ensure high productivity and performance [1]. Thus, there is a need to tap into the pool of capable young individuals who can be developed further for performance enhancements in the workforce. Attracting talents and developing them for higher positions are highly challenging for organizational management [2]. Majority of the literature, in the context of management positions, indicates that talent is "conceptualized as a code for the most effective leaders and managers at all levels, who can help a company fulfil its aspirations and drive its performance" [3]. Talent can also be viewed as referring to a limited pool of workplace individuals who possess unique competencies [4]. An employee's manifestation of skill can be used as a platform for judging whether one has a talent or just an ordinary competence in a given activity [5].

According to Rubino, healthcare is being viewed by numerous individuals as a very special type of work setting toward helping people [6]. In the case of Malaysia, healthcare organizations have a complete span of health services and they are divided into private and public organizations. Healthcare in Malaysia is primarily under the responsibility of Ministry of Health, which ensures quality healthcare through extensive range of countrywide networks of clinics and hospitals [7]. In Malaysia, upon completion of undergraduate studies, graduate medical officers need to undergo housemanship (supervised training) at identified government hospitals for 2 years [8]. In several countries, undergraduate medical education completes with housemanship. However, in Malaysia, housemanship is imposed only upon graduation in accordance with Medical Act 1971.

The term houseman refers to an advanced student or graduate in medicine obtaining supervised medical practice. In Malaysia, it is essential for doctors to undergo housemanship for 2 years after graduating with a medical degree. During the housemanship, junior doctors undergo mandatory training for 4 months in each department: emergency, medical, orthopedic, pediatrics, general surgery, anesthesia and intensive care, as well as obstetrics and gynecology [9]. The purpose of housemanship is to transform these junior doctors into medical practitioners, who are fully conversant with the treatment, types of medicines to be administered, daily necessities, workload and the complexities of the doctors' tasks. It is regarded as an essential stage in the journey of medical practitioners [10]. There is a raising concern pertaining to the disparity in the quality of junior doctors joining the medical workforce [11]. For instance, the curriculum, training and clinical exposure in various medical universities are different; the junior doctors' values and respect for a multi-ethnic, multi-cultural and multi-religious population [11] can vary with individuals. These circumstances may affect patient safety and the future of medical practice [11]. Thus, there is a need to address the issue of talent development in healthcare organizations.

Professional and medical competencies are important for junior doctors as they aid in producing competent professionals who have acquired the requisite skills, knowledge and expertise that are essential for medical practice [12]. As reported by prior researcher [13], effective talent development approach requires the existence of strong supervision and as well as talented supervisees. Specifically, it was identified that supervisory styles (participative and abusive supervisions) influence junior doctors' talent development [14]. Competence in medicine can be regarded as a latent talent that can be aroused and developed in a clinical learning environment that allows the nurturing of such innate talents [12]. Furthermore, a good clinical supervision is important toward developing an effective learning environment [15]. This implies that the junior doctors' development of professional and medical competencies (talent development) is highly dependent on the existence of strong supervision and effective repetitive experiences through exposure to a high volume of cases in clinical learning environment [15].

For a junior doctor who is undergoing housemanship, his/her accomplishment of talent development is dependent on effective supervision and through the provision of a conducive clinical learning environment [16]. A conducive clinical learning environment is termed as the atmosphere that offers social, organizational and instructional support to junior doctors in gaining knowledge from actual patients, curriculum, situation, and during individual interactions [17]. With regards to effective supervision, it has been argued that junior doctors prefer supervisors who allow participation in decision-making that promotes reciprocal and helpful work processes [18]. For instance, participative supervision stimulates a conducive clinical learning environment which leads toward developing the skills needed to be active lifelong learners throughout junior doctors' medical careers [15]. Supervisees being belittled or experiencing unfair supervisory conduct such as hostility, public criticism, and loud and angry tantrums performed by their superiors (abusive supervision) exhibit negative reactions [19]. A review of literature reveals the gap that exists in analyzing the roles of supervisory styles and clinical learning environment on the talent development of young medical professionals. This study contributes by investigating the indirect effect of clinical learning environment in the relationship between supervisory styles (participative and abusive supervisions) and talent development in the healthcare setting.

2. Theoretical and hypotheses development

A majority of the researchers pertaining to medical arena have examined the learning environment (or the immediate context of learning) based on the perspectives of experiential learning theory [15]. The experiential learning includes experiencing, observing, conceptualizing and retrying activities [20]. Experiential learning is very important for the learning process that is associated to medical arena. Prior scholar [20] posits that thoughts are not fixed, but are formed and modified throughout the acquired and prior experiences of junior doctors. These notions support the existing notions in medical field and the shift from apprentice to specialist positions [20]. Furthermore, studies pertaining to the management of expertise support the premise that supervisors play an important role in learning, particularly in providing exposure to expertise [15]. The model in this study incorporates the constructs derived from experiential learning theory which describes the supervisory styles (i.e., participative and abusive supervisions) and explains learning at work (clinical learning environment) and the development of expertise (talent development).

2.1. Indirect effect of clinical learning environment

With regards to adequate supervision for junior doctors, the contemporary learning theory stresses the "participation metaphor" (collective learning) which is termed as participative supervision [11]. Participation metaphor regards learning as a progression through participation in a collective way compared to an internal way of learning among individuals [21]. Through this approach, the individual learner becomes a member of the subject community in a gradual manner through participation in several activities in their learning arena [21].

Pertaining to healthcare environment, junior doctors recognize and value supervision approaches that support participation and engagement which are interrelated to knowledge sharing and identity formation [15]. This suggests that junior doctors can be more productive if supervisors consult junior doctors and request for opinions and recommendations to assist decision-making [6]. The perceptions within junior doctors that they are being respected and valued by their supervisors can affect junior doctors' talent development [18]. Nevertheless, as mentioned earlier, talent development among junior doctors is supported by adequate supervision and the provision of a conducive clinical learning environment [16].

A conducive clinical learning environment is an essential requirement for competent supervisees to respond to the challenges of everyday clinical practice. This is in contrast to traditional classroom approach that generates continuous development based on abstract conceptual understanding [22]. As such, it is not possible to predict or reproduce the uniqueness of real cases or the context of the clinical environment in academic environments. The junior doctors learn regularly by managing and solving the real problems of patients [23].

Talent is an individual's possession that can be enhanced through an enabling environment [5]. This reveals that supervisees feel empowered and are able to learn in an environmental and organizational system that affects their learning ability and competency management. This can be viewed according to communities of practice (COP) theory that stresses on learning compared to teaching and supported participation in practice as the central condition for junior doctors' learning [24]. The above arguments suggest that participative supervision enhances junior doctors' talent development through a conducive clinical learning environment. Thus, it could be hypothesized that:

H1: Participative style of supervision will have a positive and significant indirect effect on junior doctors' talent development through their clinical learning environment.

Prior scholars have stated that the impact of supervisor aggression is significant in understanding how workplace can reduce destructive behavior and generate an effective and productive environment for employees [25]. Supervisor aggression can be regarded as similar to abusive supervision [26]. Abusive supervision includes behaviors such as, belittling supervisees, emphasizing their shortcomings through negative evaluations, lying to supervisees, threatening, and behaving rudely to supervisees [19].

Abusive supervision has an emotional impact on supervisees at both mental and physical levels [27]. As depicted by social learning theory, supervisees impersonate the destructive behavior of their supervisor in the form of workplace [28], which depicts the relationship between destructive supervisory style (e.g., abusive supervision) and negative consequences on the supervisees. For instance, abusive supervision has been found to be associated with poor work performance and it is not likely to nurture future talent [14]. In addition, social integrationists have the view that abusive supervision may lead to supervisees being exhausted and becoming incompetent. This is because the supervisees rate their environmental quality (for instance, challenge, work control and workload) as poor compared to those who did not witness abuses in their workplace [29]. When abusive supervision takes place, the clinical learning environment becomes negative for supervisees and leads to reporting of serious medical errors by supervisees [27]. Thus, it could be hypothesized that:

H2: Abusive style of supervision will have a negative and significant indirect effect on junior doctors' talent development through their clinical learning environment.

3. Materials and methods

3.1. Data source

The study was conducted in Malaysia, one of the fastest-developing countries in South-East Asia. Junior doctors from six Malaysian public hospitals participated in this study. The hospitals are located in Klang Valley, a heavily industrialized urban area in Malaysia. Permission to carry out research in these six public hospitals was obtained from the Ethics and Research Committee of Ministry of Health Malaysia. The permission helped in gaining access to the junior doctors in these hospitals.

For this study, the sample size was computed by using the Sample Size Calculator [30]. The calculator suggested a minimum sample size of 302. A minimum required sample of 302 junior doctors from a total population of 1388 junior doctors was specifically selected from hospitals in and around the capital city of Kuala Lumpur. The sampling procedure performed was systematic sampling. Every 5th person starting from a random number of 1 to 5 was sampled (1388/302 = 4.60). In this case, since the random number is 5, the junior doctors numbered in the sequence of 5, 10, 15, 20, and so on, were sampled till reaching the required number of samples.

The questionnaires were distributed to junior doctors with the assistance of the Human Resource (HR) Training Unit at each hospital and the person in charge of the junior doctors in respective hospitals. The junior doctors were requested to send back the completed questionnaire directly to the HR Training Unit within 2 weeks from the date of distribution. Then, the completed questionnaires were personally collected from the hospitals. From the total of 450 distributed questionnaires, 355 (response rate = 79%) were completed and had tangible responses.

3.2. Measures

Measures and scales used in this study were adopted from prior literatures, which were applied and empirically tested before. The scales that were applied for each of the constructs are elaborated briefly in the following paragraphs.

3.2.1. *Participative supervision*

Participative supervision was measured using a 6-item scale [31]. Sample items for participative supervision include: "Encourages us to express ideas/suggestions" and "Uses our suggestions to make decisions that affect us," The perception of junior doctors toward the immediate supervisor's behavior in relation to participative supervision was measured using a 5-point Likert scale ranging from 1 (*Do not facilitate*) to 5 (*Highly facilitate*).

3.2.2. *Abusive supervision*

Abusive supervision scale [32] measured the non-physical aspect of abusive supervision through 15 items. Sample items for abusive supervision include: "Reminds us of our past mistakes and failures" and "Expresses anger at us when he/she is mad for another reason." In order to measure the perceptions of the junior doctors toward their immediate supervisor on abusive supervision, a 5-point rating scale that ranges from 1 (*Do not facilitate)* to 5 (*Highly facilitate)* was used.

3.2.3. *Clinical learning environment*

Clinical learning environment was measured using 10 items that were adapted from Emilia et al.'s study pertaining to the survey on junior doctors, which is based on the original version by Rotem et al. [33, 34]. This measure was applied on the aspects of environment that could facilitate talent development among junior doctors. The measurement scale for clinical learning environment was segregated into three dimensions: (1) conditions for learning (6 items), (2) general learning activities and resources (2 items) and (3) opportunities to perform rotation-specific clinical skills and assessment (2 items). Sample items for *conditions for learning* subscale include: "Extent to which we are given an appropriate level of responsibility and to carry out learning activities independently." Sample items for *general learning activities and resources* subscale include: "Extent to which learning resources and facilities were provided." Sample items for *opportunities to perform rotation-specific clinical skills and assessment* subscale include: "Extent to which we had the opportunity to practice a variety of clinical skills." The agreement of the junior doctors with the aspects of clinical learning environment was measured on a 5-point Likert scale ranging from 1 (*Do not facilitate*) to 5 (*Highly facilitate*).

3.2.4. *Talent development*

The measurement scale for talent development comprises of 13 items [35], which includes a number of competency related items representing different types of constructs of clinical and professional performances. Each item was in relation to both professional and medical competencies and computed several different aspects of an overarching competency needed by junior doctors for independent practice [30]. The main construct of professional and medical competencies was segregated into four dimensions, which include: (1) clinical competence (5 items), (2) communication competence (2 items), (3) personal competence and professional competence (6 items). Sample items for *clinical competence* subscale include: "Adequate knowledge of basic and clinical sciences and application of this knowledge." Sample items for *communication competence* subscale include: "Ability to communicate effectively and sensitively with patients and their families." Sample items for *personal and professional competence* subscale include: "Shows respect for patient autonomy and quality information sharing." Each of the items related to competencies were rated on a 5-point rating scale, ranging from 1 (*Not competent at all*) to 5 (*Highly competent).*

3.3. Pilot study

As part of the procedure to validate the questionnaire and to ensure the clarity of the items in the questionnaire, a pilot study was carried out to pre-test the questionnaire. For the purpose of this research, the questionnaire was administered randomly to a group of 30 junior doctors. These doctors were undertaking housemanship at various public hospitals in Malaysia.

3.4. Ethical considerations of the study

Toward ensuring compliance with the ethical principles, three areas were explained in the letter addressed to the hospital authorities: (1) the purpose of the study, (2) its potential benefits and (3) what is required from the junior doctors. The explanations were conveyed by providing a letter of explanation and consent form attached together with the questionnaire. The junior doctors agreed to participate by signing the attached consent form before completing the questionnaire. In order to ensure confidentiality and anonymity throughout the execution of the study, the junior doctors were not required to disclose personal information in the questionnaire.

3.5. Data analysis technique

In order to analyze the preliminary data, SPSS 22.0 was utilized. The data were then analyzed and interpreted using the SmartPLS 3 software [36], using partial least squares structural equation modelling (PLS-SEM). PLS-SEM was utilized as it is an ideal approach when the research objective is theory development and prediction oriented [37]. Furthermore, PLS is known as the family of alternating least squares algorithms that extends principal component and canonical correlation analysis [38]. Likewise SEM, in comparison with confirmatory factor analysis (CFA), extends the possibility of associations among the latent constructs and contains two elements: (1) a measurement model (essentially the CFA); and (2) a structural model [39]. A bootstrapping procedure (500 resamples) was utilized to test the significance of the *hypothesized indirect effects* which includes a 2-step procedure: (1) first, the significance of direct effect is ensured (if the significance of direct effect cannot be determined, there is no mediating effect) by utilizing bootstrapping without the presence of the mediator in the model; and (2) second, path coefficient (β), path significance (t-value) and significance of indirect effect (p-value) are examined when the mediator is integrated in the model [35]. If the significance of indirect effect cannot be determined, there is no mediating effect. Encompassing a significant indirect effect is the root to ascertain the mediator's magnitude [40].

3.6. Common method variance

Common method variance is required to be tested when data collection is carried out through self-reported questionnaires when the predictor and criterion constructs are answered by the same person [41]. As posited by prior researchers, "Invariably, when self-reported measures obtained from the same sample are utilized in research, concerns over same-source bias or general method variance arise" [42]. One of the procedures utilized to identify this issue is the Harman's single factor test, which is carried out by inserting all the principal constructs into a principal component factor analysis [43]. Proof of the appearance of method bias is when a general factor accounts for most of the covariance among the measures [41]. The findings returned an 11-factor solution with 72.7% total variance explained. The first factor accounted for only 33.93% (lower than 50%) which indicates that common method bias is not a major problem in this study.

4. Results

4.1. Assessment of measurement model

The assessment of the measurement model has the following elements: internal consistency reliability, indicator reliability, convergent validity and discriminant validity, as follows:

- Internal consistency reliability: Cronbach's alpha and composite reliability (CR) of each construct should be higher than 0.70 [44].
- Indicator reliability: Outer loadings should be higher than 0.70 [44].
- Convergent validity: The average variance extracted (AVE) should be higher than 0.50 [45, 46].
- Discriminant validity: The square root of AVE is greater than the correlations between the latent constructs [47].

Based on the assessment, the measures used within this study falls within the acceptable levels, consequently supporting the internal consistency reliability, indicator reliability, convergent validity and discriminant validity of the constructs (see **Table 1**). In addition, all of the correlations between latent constructs were below the cut-off value of 0.8, which confirms the absence of multicollinearity problems [48].

4.2. Structural model results

Upon validating the measurement model, the next stage is to examine the structural model. Multiple indicators were used to assess the quality of the structural model, [49] including the collinearity, the R^2 for exogenous-endogenous relationships, effect sizes and predictive relevance of the model [44]. To assess collinearity, variance inflation factor (VIF) values for each set of predictor constructs were calculated. As shown in **Table 2**, the VIF of all constructs was

Variable	Mean	SD	Outer loadings	Cronbach's alpha	CR	AVE	1	2	3	4
1	3.78	0.85	0.85 to 0.92	0.93	0.95	0.78	*(0.88)*			
2	2.25	1.15	0.78 to 0.92	0.98	0.98	0.77	−0.17	*(0.88)*		
3	3.85	0.73	0.79 to 0.88	0.96	0.96	0.71	0.56	−0.29	*(0.85)*	
4	3.85	0.58	0.71 to 0.84	0.92	0.94	0.62	0.30	−0.20	0.43	*(0.79)*

Italic denotes square-roots of average variance extracted (AVE) (provided within parentheses).
Legend: 1—participative supervision, 2—abusive supervision, 3—clinical learning environment, 4—talent development, SD—standard deviation, CR—composite reliability, and AVE—average variance extracted.

Table 1. Measurement model results.

Predictor variables	Dependent variables	
	3	4
	VIF	VIF
1	1.03	1.47
2	1.03	1.09
3		1.55

Legend: (1) participative supervision, (2) abusive supervision, (3) clinical learning environment, (4) talent development, VIF—variance inflation factor.

Table 2. Collinearity assessment.

below 5.0, which indicates that the level of collinearity is low [44]. To evaluate the structural models' predictive power, R^2 was calculated. R^2 denotes the total of variance explained by the exogenous constructs [50]. All three constructs together explained 20.1% of the variance, which demonstrates moderate predictive power [51].

The effect size f^2 assesses an exogenous construct's contribution to an endogenous latent construct's R^2 value. The f^2 values of 0.02, 0.15, and 0.35 reveal an exogenous construct's small, medium, or large effect, respectively [44]. In this path model, the exogenous constructs participative supervision, abusive supervision, clinical learning environment for explaining the endogenous latent construct talent development has effect size of 0.106, which reflects the small to medium effect of these factors on talent development. Finally, the predictive accuracy, Q^2, of the model was assessed using the blindfolding procedure. The resulting Q^2 value of talent development is 0.12. The Q^2 value is larger than 0, which reveals that the model is within the acceptable fit for predictive relevance [44].

4.3. Assessing the indirect effect of clinical learning environment

In order to test the indirect effect of clinical learning environment, the respective construct (clinical learning environment) was removed from the model. The direct path coefficients from (1) participative supervision to talent development ($\beta = 0.28$, $t = 4.68$, $p = 0.000$) and (2) abusive supervision to talent development (β = −0.16, t = 3.01, p = 0.000) in the absence of a clinical learning environment were significant. Bootstrapping procedure [52] was utilized to test the indirect paths from participative supervision to talent development and abusive supervision to talent development. The indirect effects of (1) participative supervision on talent development (β = 0.19, t = 4.28, p = 0.000) and (2) abusive supervision on talent development (β = −0.07, t = 3.16, p = 0.002) mediated by clinical learning environment were significant. Thus, this indicates that hypotheses H1 and H2 were supported. The summary of findings is illustrated in **Figure 1**.

After confirming the significance of indirect effects by bootstrapping, variance accounted for (VAF) was computed [44]. The VAF determines the size of the indirect effect in relation to the total effect (i.e., direct effect + indirect effect). VAF is calculated as a proportion of total effect (VAF = indirect effect/total effect). The VAF values of 0.69 (68.81%; greater than 20% and less than 80%) and 0.46 (45.81%; greater than 20% and less than 80%) indicate that clinical learning environment partially mediates the relationship between (1) participative supervision

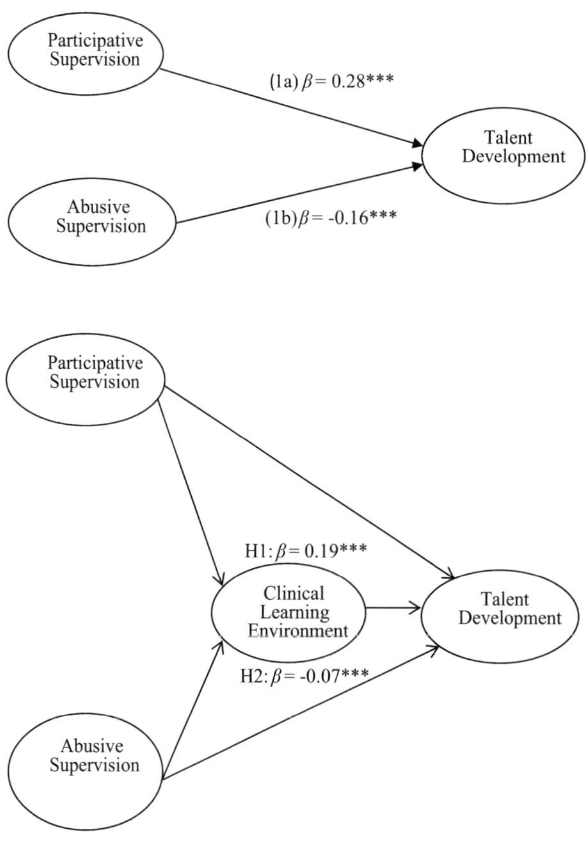

Figure 1. Direct and indirect model. Legend: (1a) and (1b) = Value without the intervening construct; ***significant at level p = 0.001.

and talent development and (2) abusive supervision and talent development. In other words, the influence of participative and abusive supervision on talent development partially affects clinical learning environment and then, in turn, affects talent development.

5. Discussion

The findings demonstrate a significant indirect effect of clinical learning environment on the participative supervision-talent development and abusive supervision-talent development links. In general, the result of this study is consistent with prior scholars who asserted that clinical learning environment indirectly affects the relationship between participative supervision and talent development [15, 53, 54]. Participative supervision through a conducive clinical learning environment plays an important role in enhancing junior doctors' development of professional and medical competencies [15]. This finding suggests that junior doctors should be provided opportunities to establish their competencies by allowing them to participate in on-the-job decisions in the clinical environment. A conducive clinical learning environment that allows empowerment can lead to development of competencies such as clinical, communication, professional and medical. The junior doctors should be allowed to learn from errors committed by them and the errors made by others. The supervisors of junior doctors should infuse confidence among their supervisees' so that the junior doctors can carry out their work and generate appropriate method to formulate decisions on the job when the supervisor is not present in the department. As the junior doctors are closest to the details, the decisions made by them can be better than decisions made by their supervisors.

This result is in line with previous studies to predict abusive supervision is a determinant of clinical environment in influencing junior doctors' talent development (development of professional and medical competencies). According to Carl Rogers who pioneered theories on counseling, believes in an environment in which individuals are able to express themselves in an open manner [55]. Consequently, such an uncritical environment encourages confidence in the supervisee as they feel free to explore new knowledge without fear of reproach [55]. Thus, a good learning environment is one in which the junior will not be frightened to ask questions for fear of being criticized and reprimanded [56]. In contrast, an under-resourced clinical environment with inadequate infrastructure or personnel (1) impedes junior doctors' accomplishment of clinical tasks [57], (2) impacts patient safety [27], and (3) is associated with serious medical errors [58, 59]. It is clear that abusive supervision influences junior doctors' turnover intention through an unconducive clinical learning environment. Thus, junior doctors who feel abused have reduced capacity to work and participate in the learning environment, which consequently affect the junior doctors' talent development (development of professional and medical competencies).

5.1. Theoretical implications

The empirical evidence on the indirect effect of clinical learning environment on the relationship between supervisory styles (participative and abusive supervisions) and junior doctors' talent development is an essential theoretical contribution of this study. In other words, this study enhances our understanding about potential underlying mechanisms that are responsible for the relationship between the supervisory styles (participative and abusive supervisions) and talent development among junior doctors. The findings herein confirm that participative supervision through a conducive clinical learning environment plays an important role in enhancing junior doctors' talent development. Thus, a conducive clinical learning environment that allows empowerment leads to talent development. The abusive supervision is a determinant of clinical environment in influencing junior doctors' talent development. The junior doctors who feel abused have reduced capacity to work and participate in the learning environment which consequently affects their talent development.

5.2. Practical implications

This study also offers practical implications. The finding of this study indicates that participative supervision influences talent development of public hospital junior doctors through a conducive clinical learning environment. Thus, public hospital administrators should provide opportunities for junior doctors to develop real-time professional experiences, including applying their skills and enhancing their professional and medical competencies in a clinical environment. For instance, administrators can build up junior doctors' professional and medical skills through participative supervision and problem solving activities.

The findings of this study also indicate that abusive supervision indirectly affects talent development in the presence of clinical learning environment. It shows the need to provide a conducive environment to junior doctors at public hospitals to nurture and enhance their ability to professional and medical competencies. Public hospital administrators should execute training programs that can support junior doctors in developing their professional and medical competencies. For instance, junior doctors could be trained to challenge the situation and become confident in facing the negative consequences in their learning environment. Furthermore, public hospital administrators should provide a grievance system [60] to prevent supervisors' abusive behavior that may occur during the housemanship training.

The administrators of public hospitals can develop programs to train immediate senior medical officers and specialists (supervisors) to be aware of their interactions with the junior doctors (supervisees). Immediate senior medical officers and specialists should be warned that abusive supervision will have harmful effects on junior doctors. Additionally, by providing a conducive clinical learning environment which involves increasing junior doctors' associations with patients and colleagues, the workplace will be able to increase the competencies of supervisees.

Overall, the result of this study demonstrates that conducive clinical learning environment is critically important for junior doctors to have effective housemanship learning and training processes. These findings have identified some interesting views on the supervisors' role that may be possible to apply to hospital settings. For instance, supervisors have the responsibility of designing the learning conditions that provide sufficient structure and support to optimize junior doctors' learning. The amount of structure and assistance offered should vary based on the developmental level of the junior doctors [61]. The supervisor's assessment of the developmental level of the junior doctors will aid in identifying the type of learning environment that is optimal for training. Furthermore, public hospital administrators can develop training modules relative to the needs of junior doctors and generate an environment that will encourage the junior doctors to manage their professional and medical competencies.

6. Limitations and directions for future research

This study has a few limitations. The first limitation is the cross-sectional character of this study. As such, a longitudinal model can be carried out to further explore the links among participative supervision, abusive supervision, clinical learning environment and talent development. The second limitation is the small percentage of explained variances on the talent development of junior doctors. As mentioned before, the model explained 20.1% of the variance in talent development. The small percentage of explained variances of junior doctors' talent development could be related to other constructs apart from the studied ones. Again, this particular gap can be further explored. Third, the study samples herein are restricted to public hospital junior doctors only. Therefore, caution must be taken in applying the results outside of this spectrum. For example, precautions need to be taken in generalizing the findings of this study to the private hospitals as well. Thus, future research can consider junior doctors from the private hospitals to generalize and harmonize the present findings. A comparison study involving both public and private hospital junior doctors can be undertaken to confirm the associations between the constructs and justify the dissimilarities, if any.

7. Conclusion

In particular, the result of this study is consistent with theoretical propositions that clinical learning environment indirectly affects the relationship between participative supervision-talent development and abusive supervision-talent development. This study contributes to the clinical learning environment literature by providing empirical support toward identifying clinical learning environment as the underlying mechanism that accounts for the participative supervision-talent development and abusive supervision-talent development relationships. Finally, it is hoped that this study will induce and trigger more research interests in this field for future researches.

Acknowledgements

The authors thank the authorities of the public hospitals and the junior doctors who participated in the study. The authors also thank the Ministry of Health, Malaysia, for giving consent to conduct the study.

Author details

Anusuiya Subramaniam[1]*, Murali Sambasivan[2] and Abu Daud Silong[3]

*Address all correspondence to: anusuiya.vs@gmail.com

1 Faculty of Business and Management, Asia Pacific University of Technology and Innovation (APU), Technology Park Malaysia, Bukit Jalil, Kuala Lumpur, Malaysia

2 Taylor's Business School, Taylor's University Lakeside Campus, Subang Jaya, Selangor, Malaysia

3 Universiti Putra Malaysia, Serdang, Selangor, Malaysia

References

[1] Evangelou CE, Karacapidilis N. A multidisciplinary approach for supporting knowledge-based decision making in collaborative settings. International Journal on Artificial Intelligence Tools. 2007;**16**(6):1069-1092

[2] Abdul Hamid Z, Osman-Gani AM. Contemporary issues in human resource development. In: Human Resource Development in Malaysia. Malaysia: Pearson; 2011. pp. 303-333. Available from: http://irep.iium.edu.my/11165/ [Accessed: 29-07-2012]

[3] Michaels E, Handfield-Jones H, Axelrod B. The War for Talents. Watertown, MA: Harvard Business School Press; 2001

[4] Garavan TN, Carbery R, Rock A. Mapping talent development: Definition, scope and architecture. European Journal of Training and Development. 2012;**36**(1):5-24

[5] Kabwe CB. The Conceptualisation and Operationalisation of Talent Management: The Case of European Internationally Operating Businesses. 2011. Available from: http://clok.uclan.ac.uk/2812 /3/Kabwe_Chitalu_Final_e-Thesis_%28Master_Copy%29.pdf [Accessed: 31-12-2013]

[6] Rubino L. Leadership. In: Buchbinder SB, Shanks NH, editors. Introduction to Health Care Management. Sudbury, MA: Jones & Bartlett Publishers; 2011. pp. 17-38

[7] Lee S. Disaster management and emergency medicine in Malaysia. The Western Journal of Emergency Medicine. 2011;**12**(1). Available from: http://escholarship.org/uc/item/9gv4h27b) [Accessed: 15-06-2012]

[8] Overworked Housemen. 2011. Available from: http://www.thesundaily.my/news/167606 [Accessed: 11-05-2012]

[9] Bedi RS, Azizan H. 2008. Young Docs Walk a Tightrope. Available from: http://intan-frenny.blogspot.com/2010/03/housemanship-in-malaysia.html [Accessed: 06-01-2013]

[10] Yusoff MS, Tan YJ, Esa AR. Stress, stressors and coping strategies among house officers in a Malaysian hospital. ASEAN. Journal of Psychiatry. 2011;**12**(1):85-94

[11] Lum M. 2016. The Dilemma of Training Young Doctors. Available from: http://www.star2.com/living/viewpoints/2016/08/28/the-dilemma-of-training-young-doctors/ [Accessed: 13-10-2017]

[12] Adewale AA, Manaf NHA, Omar A. Competence in medical practice as perceived by malaysian medical interns: A measurement invariance analysis. Journal of Education and Vocational Research. 2012;**3**(7):225-233

[13] Lockwood NR. Talent management driver for organizational success. HR Magazine. 2006;**51**(6):1-11

[14] Ayree S, Chen ZX, Sun L, Debrah YA. Antecedents and outcomes of abusive supervision: Test of a trickle-down model. The Journal of Applied Psychology. 2007;**92**(1):191-201

[15] Sheehan DC. Learning and supervision in internship: A sociocultural framework for framework for understanding learning and supervision in medical internship. 2011. Available from: http://ir.canterbury.ac.nz/bitstream/10092/5350/1/Thesis_fulltext.pdf [Accessed on 31-10-2013]

[16] Bleakley A. Pre-registration house officers and ward-based learning "a new apprenticeship" model. Medical Education. 2002;**36**(1):9-15

[17] Dornan T, Muijtjens A, Graham J, Scherpbier A, Boshuizen H. Manchester clinical placement index (MCPI): Conditions for medical students' learning in hospital and community placements. Advances in Health Sciences Education. 2012;**17**(5):703-716

[18] Sullivan EJ, Decker PJ. Effective Leadership and Management in Nursing. 7th ed. Prentice Hall: Upper Saddle River, NJ; 2009

[19] Gregory BT, Osmonbekov T, Gregory ST, Albritton MD, Carr JC. Abusive supervision and citizenship behaviors: Exploring boundary conditions. Journal of Managerial Psychology. 2012;**28**(6):628-644

[20] Kolb DA. Experiential Learning: Experience as the Source of Learning and Development. Prentice–Hall: Englewood-Cliffs, NJ; 1984

[21] Sfard A. On two metaphors for learning and the dangers of choosing just one. Educational Researcher. 1998;**27**(2):4-13

[22] Beirne M, Knight S. From community theatre to critical management studies. Management Learning. 2007;**38**(5):591-611

[23] Teunissen PW, Scheele F, Scherpbier AJ, Van Der Vleuten CPM, Boor K, Van Luijk SJ. Van Diemen-Steenvoorde JA.: (2007) how residences learn: Qualitative evidence for the pivotal role of clinical activities. Medical Education. 2007;**41**(8):763-770

[24] Dornan T, Mann K, Scherpbier A, Spencer J. Introduction. In: Dornan T, Mann K, Scherpbier A, Spencer J, editors. Medical Education. Theory and Practice. Churchill Livingstome: Edinburgh; 2011

[25] Mitchell MS, Ambrose ML. Employees' behavioral reactions to supervisor aggression: An examination of individual and situational factors. The Journal of Applied Psychology. 2012;**97**(6):1148-1170

[26] Tepper BJ. Abusive supervision in work organizations: Review, synthesis, and research agenda. Journal of Management. 2007;**33**(3):261-289

[27] Launer J. Bullying in the health service. Postgraduate Medical Journal. 2013;**89**(1051): 294-304

[28] Schyns B, Schilling J. How bad are the effects of bad leaders? A meta-analysis of destructive leadership and its outcomes. The Leadership Quarterly. 2013;**24**(1):138-158

[29] Ahmer S, Yousafzai AW, Bhutto N, Alam S, Sarangzai AK, Iqbal A. Bullying of medical students in Pakistan: A cross-sectional questionnaire survey. PLoS One. 2008;**3**(12):e3889. DOI: 10.1371/journal.pone.0003889

[30] Sample Size Calculator. 2004. Available from: http://www.raosoft.com/samplesize.html. [Accessed: 20-03-2013]

[31] Arnold JA, Arad S, Rhoades JA, Drasgow F. The empowering leadership questionnaire: The construction and validation of a new scale for measuring leader behaviors. Journal of Organizational Behavior. 2000;**21**(3):249-269

[32] Tepper BJ. Consequences of abusive supervision. Academy of Management Journal. 2000;**43**(2):178-190

[33] Emilia O, Bloomfield L, Rotem A. Replication of a clinical learning environment survey for junior medical officers: A study of medical students in an Indonesian hospital. Focus on Health Professional Education: A Multi-Disciplinary Journal. 2006;**7**(3):36-47

[34] Rotem A, Godwin P, Du J. Learning in hospital settings. Teaching and Learning in Medicine. 1995;**7**(4):211-217

[35] McGill DA, Van Der Vleuten CPM, Clarke MJ. A critical evaluation of the validity and the reliability of global competency constructs for supervisor assessment of junior medical trainees. Advances in Health Sciences Education. 2013;**18**(4):701-725

[36] Ringle CM, Wende S, Becker JM. SmartPLS 3. Bönningstedt: SmartPLS; 2015. Available from: http://www.smartpls.com. [Accessed 2016-06-31]

[37] Hair JF, Ringle CM, Sarstedt M. PLS-SEM: Indeed a silver bullet. Journal of Marketing Theory and Practice. 2011;**19**(2):139-151

[38] Henseler J, Sarstedt M. Goodness-of-fit indices for partial least squares path modeling. Computational Statistics. 2012;**28**(2):565-580

[39] Schreiber JB, Nora A, Stage FK, Barlow EA, King J. Reporting structural equation modeling and confirmatory factor analysis results: A review. The Journal of Educational Research. 2006;**99**(6):323-337

[40] Preacher KJ, Hayes AF. Asymptotic and resampling strategies for assessing and comparing indirect effects in multiple mediator models. Behavior Research Methods. 2008;**40**(3):879-891

[41] Podsakoff PM, MacKenzie SB, Lee J, Podsakoff NP. Common method biases in behavioral research: A critical review of the literature and recommended remedies. The Journal of Applied Psychology. 2003;**88**(5):879-903

[42] Podsakoff PM, Todor WD. Relationships between leader reward and punishment behavior and and group processes and productivity. Journal of Management. 1985;**11**(1):55-73

[43] Podsakoff P, Organ D. Self-reports in organizational research: Problems and prospects. Journal of Management. 1986;**12**(4):531-543

[44] Hair JF, Hult GTM, Ringle CM, Sarstedt M. A Primer on Partial Least Squares Structural Equation Modeling (PLS-SEM). Thousand Oaks, CA: Sage Publications; 2014

[45] Chin W. Issues and opinion on structural equation modelling. MIS Quarterly. 1998;**22**(1):7-16

[46] Hair JF Jr, Anderson RE, Tatham RL, Black WC. Multivariate Data Analysis. 5th ed. Porto Alegre: Bookman; 2005

[47] Fornell C, Larcker DF. Evaluating structural equation models with unobservable variables and measurement error. Journal of Marketing Research. 1981;**18**(1):39-50

[48] Bryman A, Cramer D. Quantitative Data Analysis for Social Scientists. New York, NY: Routledge; 1994

[49] O'Cass A. Political advertising believability and information source value during elections. Journal of Advertising. 2002;**31**(1):63-74

[50] Barclay D, Higgins C, Thompson R. The partial least squares (PLS) approach to causal modelling: Personal computer adoption and use as an illustration. Technology Studies. 1995;**2**(2):285-309

[51] Cohen J. Statistical Power Analysis for the Behavioural Sciences. Hillsdale, New Jersey: Lawrence Erlbaum Associates; 1988

[52] MacKinnon DP. Introduction to Statistical Mediation Analysis. Mahwah, NJ: Erlbaum; 2008

[53] Billett S. Towards a workplace pedagogy: Guidance, participation and engagement. Adult Education Quarterly. 2002;**53**(1):27-43

[54] Henderson A, Twentyman M, Heel A, Lloyd B. Students' perception of the psycho-social clinical learning environment: An evaluation of placement models. Nurse Education Today. 2006;**26**(7):564-571

[55] Walsh D. The Nurse Mentor's Handbook: Supporting Students in Clinical Practice. Berkshire: Open University Press; 2010

[56] Gourevitch MN, Malaspina D, Weitzman M, Goldfrank LR. The public hospital in American medical education. Journal of Urban Health. 2008;**85**(5):779-786

[57] Hauer KE, Ten Cate O, Boscardin C, Irby DM, Iobst W, O'Sullivan PS. Understanding trust as an essential element of trainee supervision and learning in the workplace. Advances in Health Sciences Education. 2014;**19**(3):435-456

[58] Imran N, Jawaid M, Haider II, Masood Z. Bullying of junior doctors in Pakistan: A cross-sectional survey. Singapore Medical Journal. 2010;**51**(7):592-595

[59] Paice E, Smith D. Bullying of trainee doctors is a patient safety issue. The Clinical Teacher. 2009;**6**(1):13-17

[60] Boswell WR, Olson-Buchanan JB. Experiencing mistreatment at work: The role of grievance filing, nature of mistreatment, and employee withdrawal. Academy of Management Journal. 2004;**47**(1):129-139

[61] Austin DR. Therapeutic Recreation: Processes and Techniques. 5th ed. Champaign, IL: Sagamore Publishing; 2004

Chapter 3

Change Management Support in Postgraduate Medical Education: A Change for the Better

Lindsay Bank, Mariëlle Jippes,
Albert J.J.A. Scherpbier and Fedde Scheele

Additional information is available at the end of the chapter

http://dx.doi.org/10.5772/intechopen.72113

Abstract

Curriculum change is inevitably a part of postgraduate medical education (PGME) due to a necessity to rapidly adapt to changes in societal needs, educational philosophy and technological advances. Initiating, adopting as well as sustaining successful change can be very challenging especially in complex and time-constrained environments such as healthcare and PGME. Indeed, research has shown that educational changes do not always lead to the desired adjustments in practice. Surprisingly, implementation processes in healthcare and, more particularly, those in medical education are rarely supported by change management principles despite the scale and implications of curriculum reforms that justify guidance of such implementation processes. Insights from a change management perspective could help to smoothen the transition from theory to practice by guiding implementation processes and provide support in routinizing innovations in standard practice. A thorough description about change from an educational as well as a change management perspective is made, followed by the experiences with introducing change management principles into PGME. Lastly, the potential of change management principles for future changes in medical education, and their practical implications, is presented.

Keywords: change management, postgraduate medical education, curriculum change, readiness for change, innovation

1. Introduction

Change and learning happen throughout our lives as we need to adapt to the world around us [1]. Change and innovation imply progress and improvement from our current state of practice to a desired state of practice. Change creates new opportunities as well as new demands on our way of behaving and the goals we need to achieve. This implies that we need to learn to change. Learning in itself brings about change as well when you acquire new capabilities and skills which create new opportunities and choices leading to further growth, and inevitably change [1]. However, change can be challenging as it disturbs an equilibrium before reaching a new, and presumably improved, one [2]. Change is a continuous process, and it is only a matter of time before a new equilibrium is sought.

1.1. Change management in postgraduate medical education

As mentioned above, change or innovation implies progress and improvement. This presumption is clearly reflected in healthcare policy in which innovation is used among others to increase efficiency, reduce costs, raise patient satisfaction, reduce practice variation and improve quality [3, 4]. And of course, with time, innovations become outdated themselves and need to be replaced or adapted [3]. The same trend is seen in education. Medical education needs to adapt to among others technological advances, societal demands and legislation. As a result, new methods of teaching and learning are introduced or current methods are adapted [5–8].

Despite the fact that implementing change is notoriously challenging, support from a change management perspective to support implementation processes in postgraduate medical education (PGME) is still rarely sought [9]. This might be the result of a strong disciplinary divide between management sciences and health or educational sciences. Indeed, when looking at the literature, authors of studies with primary relevance to implementation science typically publish almost exclusively in management literature [10]. This slows the spread of innovation because it stifles the extent to which research evidence for change purposes is sought, exchanged and applied [11, 12]. Attention to change management principles in healthcare and educational settings is also important to avoid the use of inappropriate, ineffective strategies for implementation and hence save time and money [13]. Too little guidance from appropriate change models and implementation strategies could slow down the implementation process, mainly because opportunities for advanced assessment and planning are missed [14–16]. Additionally, change management principles can provide methods to perform formative evaluations of the implementation process; so, change efforts can be optimized, and sustainability of the innovation can be prolonged and potentially promote dissemination of findings to other contexts [17].

1.2. Reading guide

In this chapter, a thorough description about change from an educational as well as a change management perspective is made. Insights from, among others, the diffusion of innovation theory by Rogers [18] as well as the three-stage model of change by Lewin [2] are used to discuss the challenges of change implementation in general. This is followed by an extensive explanation of the factors involved in implementing change in medical education such as complex systems, diverse educational contexts, culture as well as the influence of the medical profession itself. The potential of change management in PGME is discussed based on empirical research [9, 16, 19]. Lastly, practical implications are presented.

2. The challenge of implementing change

For decades, the study of change has been one of the important research topics in the social sciences because implementing change has proven to be difficult and success rates are disappointing [4, 20, 21]. Organizational change is particularly challenging as it requires multiple, usually simultaneous, adjustments in workflow, communication, decision-making and so on. In other words, it requires collective and coordinated behavioral change [4]. Not surprisingly, it is said that more than 50% of organizational change attempts eventually or prematurely fail [4, 21, 22]. There is no reason to believe the numbers are any better for change processes in healthcare organizations [4]. For instance, when looking at the implementation of new treatment methods and guidelines into routine practice, indeed this proves to be a slow and unpredictable process [3, 23]. Many interventions found to be effective in research settings fail to translate into the expected patient care outcomes in real practice [17]. Furthermore, medical innovations tend to be added to the already existing repertoire of diagnostic or therapeutic options rather than replacing them. The latter makes the life cycles of medical innovations relatively long [24].

2.1. Adopting change

In his diffusion of innovation theory, Rogers argues people tend to adopt changes at varying rates. Adoption of an innovation is an individual process detailing the series of stages one undergoes from first hearing about a change to finally adopting it. Rogers identifies five adopter categories, or classification of members of a social system, on the basis of their innovativeness. Innovativeness is the extent to which an individual is relatively early in adopting new ideas. Their relative speeds can be plotted as a normal distribution, showing the incidence of people adopting an innovation at various points in time [18]. The normal curve (**Figure 1**) is used to delineate five different categories of adopters according to where they fall under the curve: innovators (2.5%), early adopters (13.5%), early majority (34%), late majority (34%) and laggards (16%) [18]. These five categories of adopters have the following characteristics [18].

- *Innovators* are the first to adopt an innovation. They are eager to try new ideas and willing to accept a setback when an idea proves unsuccessful. Others might consider the innovator to be daring, and it is the hazardous risk-taking that is of salient value to this type of individual.
- *Early adopters* seem to have the greatest degree of opinion leadership. They provide advice and information sought by other adopters. The early adopter is usually respected by his or her peers and has a reputation for successful and discrete use of new ideas.
- *Early majority* adopt new ideas just before the average member of a social system. They deliberate some time before completely adopting a new idea. Seldom leading, early majority adopters willingly follow in adopting innovations.
- *Late majority* are skeptical. Their adoption may be borne out of economic necessity and in response to increasing social pressure. They are cautious about innovations and are reluctant to adopt until most others in their social system do so first.

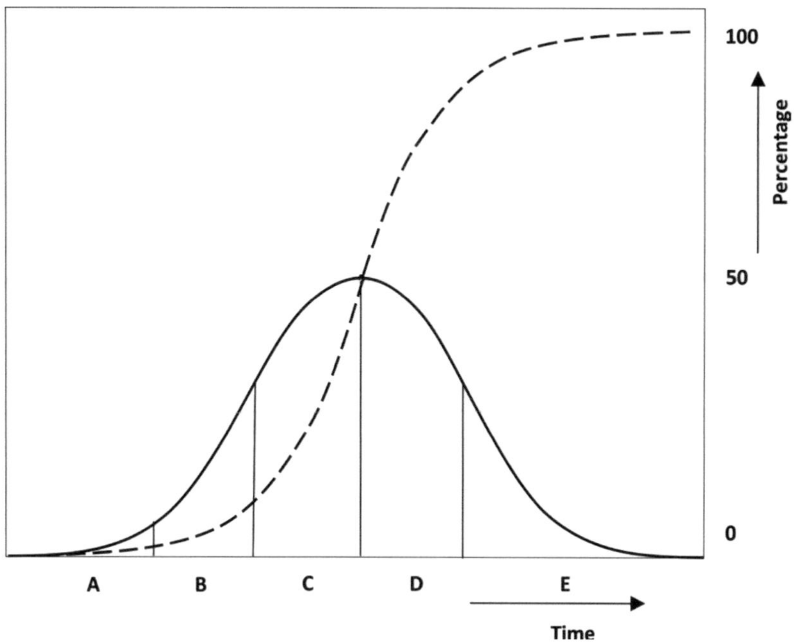

Figure 1. Diffusion of innovation. The figure shows the normal curve (black line) representing the different adopter types identified by Rogers and the S-curve (dashed line) showing the cumulative percentage, or prevalence, of people adopting an innovation at various points in time. Adopter categories: (A) innovators, (B) early adopters, (C) early majority, (D) late majority and (E) laggards.

- *Laggards* are traditionalists and possess almost no opinion leadership. Innovation finally adopted by a laggard may already be rendered obsolete by more recent ideas already in use by innovators.

In addition to the characteristics of the adopters, the perceived characteristics of an innovation are also considered to affect its adoption and diffusion. Whereas adoption refers to an individual process, diffusion signifies a group phenomenon. Diffusion suggests how an innovation spreads and can be plotted as an S-curve showing the cumulative percentage, or prevalence, of people adopting an innovation at various points in time (**Figure 1**). Rogers identifies five innovation attributes as being important for rapid diffusion [18]:

1. Relative advantage, that is, the degree to which the innovation is perceived to have significant advantages over current practice such as higher productivity, efficiency and lower costs.
2. Compatibility, that is, the degree to which the innovation is perceived as being consistent with past practices, current values and existing needs of potential adopters.
3. Complexity, that is, the degree to which the innovation can be readily understood and easily implemented.
4. Trialability, that is, the degree to which the innovation may be experimented with or tried out, within certain limits, before actually adopting the innovation.
5. Observability, that is, the degree to which the use and benefits of the innovation are visible to others and as a consequence can act as a stimulus for uptake by others.

However, it is important to realize that adoption of an innovation does not mean exact replication. In the process of adoption and implementation of an innovation, it can be adapted or reinvented. Reinvention is defined as the degree to which an innovation is changed or modified in the process of its adoption and implementation. Reinvention is a key principle in Diffusion of Innovation. The success of an innovation depends on how well it evolves to meet the needs of more and more risk-averse individuals. For instance, reinvention is likely to occur in the case of complex innovations or when an innovation has multiple applications. Alternatively, reinvention can also occur when adopters lack sufficient knowledge about the innovation or when the innovation is an abstract concept leading to uncertainties. The concept of reinvention is important because it tells us that continuous improvement of an innovation is the key to its diffusion [18].

3. Implementation of change in medical education

In the last decade, the most prominent change PGME faced was the introduction of competency based medical education (CBME). This innovation is driven by, among others, changes in healthcare needs and expectations of the public [25, 26] as well as a need to show a greater accountability to society [27]. Increasingly, medicine is being asked to be receptive as well as reactive to societal needs and be conscious about the outcomes of their educational programs [26, 27]. Not surprisingly, competency-based frameworks are designed to be outcome-oriented: they focus on competencies needed by trainees at the end of their training in order to meet the healthcare needs of society [26]. To reach this goal, CBME introduced a broader definition of competencies [26] as well as requirements for teaching and assessment strategies [25]. For instance, in the case of CanMEDS, this means trainees also need to become a competent 'leader,' 'collaborator' and 'scholar.'

The introduction of an outcome-based framework led to a cascade of changes such as the development of so called entrustable professional activities (EPAs [28]) and increased use of portfolios. For the purpose of constructing competency-based PGME, activities that constitute elements of professional work may be specified to a limited number of EPAs. EPAs are 'those activities that together constitute the mass of critical elements that operationally define a profession.' EPAs should be considered as units of work that have been specified with a number of conditions to be met in order to receive a statement of awarded responsibility (STAR) [28]. For instance, obstetric EPAs include technical activities such as preforming a cesarean section as well as more generic ones such as delivering bad news. A STAR for a specific EPA marks to what extend a trainee is entrusted to carry out this activity independently [28]. CBME and EPAs emphasized the role of assessment and created a need to properly organize assessment information. To support competency development in PGME, the use of portfolios is increased to manage the large volume of assessment data collected. The uptake of portfolios was further driven by their potential to promote a trainee's active engagement in and responsibility for learning as well as endorsement of regulatory bodies [29].

Altogether, these changes in PGME ask for a paradigm shift [25, 26] from a focus solely on reaching medical expertise to a focus on becoming a medical expert as well as acquiring other competencies for trainees to successfully address the roles they have in meeting societal needs.

In other words, the theoretical changes require behavioral changes of individuals, in this case medical specialists and trainees. In practice, this means purposeful deliberate activity from supervising medical specialists to ensure proper use of feedback and reflection on learning [29].

However, implementing change is easier said than done especially in time-constrained environments such as healthcare and PGME. Challenges in the implementation process of CBME lead back to generic models for CBME that are not always specifically outlined. This results in a lack of clarity about its content, meaning and relevance [5, 30, 31]. Furthermore, the implementation of CBME frameworks is further complicated by a lack of support from educationalists who can help with understanding the educational concepts and relating them to the clinical work place [14, 25]. From an educationalist's point of view, learning objectives must be specified and there is a tendency to split each of these objectives in more detail. Indeed, this has been done in the Accreditation Council of Graduate Medical Education (ACGME) and CanMEDS frameworks. In practice, however, medical specialists have no problem stating which professional activities need to be carried out adequately by their trainees at which moment in time but they have trouble valuing these activities as competencies [28].

Additionally, innovation in medical education must compete with other goals of healthcare such as efficiency and coverage. When translating this to the introduction of outcome-based learning, this raises questions such as 'how can we ensure more direct observation of the trainee during busy consultation hours?'; 'how do we deal with uncertain timings of transitions?' and 'how do we ensure faculty development?' [32]. In the complex dynamics of a teaching hospital, clinical service and medical education are interrelated. This means that changes in medical education change the context of clinical service and vice versa [33].

3.1. Complex organizations

Due to this intricate balance between the different goals of a teaching hospital, complexity theory has recently gained attention in educational research. Complexity theory approaches an organization as a set of subsystems. These subsystems are connected to each other and have to be analyzed in the context of, and in relation to, other systems rather than in isolation [33–35]. In teaching hospitals, PGME and clinical service are so tightly embedded that changes to one of these systsems immediately have an effect on the other. This frequently leads to friction between systems [33–35]. For instance, CBME has led to the introduction of flexible training programs that can no longer be modeled around clinical service [34]. The early departure of a highly talented trainee competent enough to speed up his/her progression through the training program, may have workforce implications and impact on healthcare as trainee schedules are disrupted [32].

Complex systems also have fuzzy boundaries, meaning that these systems are not always clearly defined [33, 34]. People working in these systems might have several roles in multiple systems as well. For example, a gynecologist performing a cesarean section delivers patient care, educates a trainee and acts as a manager in the operating room. Additionally, complex systems often behave in a nonlinear way. This means that change in one system can lead to unintentional, unpredicted and disproportional effects and outcomes in another system. This makes complex systems sensitive to small changes [3, 33, 34]. As a result, the implementation process cannot be completely preprogrammed [3] and needs to be adaptable.

3.2. Implementation in different educational contexts

Competency-based frameworks are introduced in many areas of the world [5–8, 25]. As a result, these theoretical frameworks need to be translated to many different contexts. Starting of small, even within one country, implementing the same innovation at different teaching sites can be challenging. For instance, program objectives are usually centrally set but must be achieved at local teaching sites. As a result, these individual teaching sites must adapt to meet these objectives [29], which might not always be possible due to their local context such as the lack of certain treatment facilities. Diversity in curriculum structures across teaching sites such as longitudinal programs versus rotation-based programs could also bring forward other needs when implementing the same change [29].

Organizational characteristics of the teaching site itself, such as their size, might influence the implementation process as well. For instance, in the Netherlands, larger academic medical teaching centers tend to be less receptive for change compared to the smaller nonacademic teaching hospital [16]. Departments are usually smaller in nonacademic teaching hospitals, which might lead to more efficient communication and decision-making processes [14]. Possibly, it might also cause team members to feel a stronger sense of a shared responsibility for educational change [14], thus promoting teamwork when implementing change [16]. Additionally, the primary focus in academic medical teaching hospitals tends to be more on pursuing an active career in research rather than an active career in medical education [36–39]. Potentially, this could impede gaining sufficient support and shared efforts to implement educational change [16].

Innovation can also be translated to another educational context. Initially, competency frameworks were developed for postgraduate medical education, but they are increasingly translated to undergraduate medical education as well. This requires the competencies to be related to the another professional environment in which they must be achieved [28].

In the case of competency-based frameworks, they are developed in different countries [40, 41] and are being used to guide the design of medical curricula all over the world [5, 25, 27, 30]. Due to the differences in health and educational systems, some elements of these frameworks might be variously executable in different countries. As a result, minor adjustments to the framework might be necessary in order for it to fit into other contexts [42]. In this case, every country has the freedom to make these adjustments. However, it becomes more complex when you intend to implement a curriculum that is intended to be applied across borders, such as a pan-European curriculum in PGME [42]. In that case, you set a certain standard that needs to be met by all countries involved. As a consequence, such a curriculum must respect local practice variation while providing a standard set of outcomes, duration and subjects of training. One way of achieving that would be to create a mandatory core for all trainees as well as complementary electives. The latter allows variation between both personal and local needs and infrastructure [42].

3.3. The influence of organizational culture on curriculum change

Not surprisingly, within these different educational settings, the influence of culture is widely acknowledged to be important for innovation [43–47]. Organizational culture is defined as a set of beliefs, values and assumptions that are shared by members of an organization [48]. Organizational members rely on these values and beliefs to guide their decisions and behaviors

[44, 48]. Organizational culture can differ between countries and between organizations within countries, and it can even vary between departments within the same organization. Therefore, being aware of or even assessing the culture of these individual departments is essential for the successful implementation of change [44].

The competing values framework developed by Quinn et al. [49] explores competing demands within an organization on two axes. Organizations are classified according to whether they value flexibility or control in organizational structuring and whether they adopt an internal or external focus toward the environment. This leads to the four possible culture types, that is, 'human relations,' 'open systems,' 'internal process' and 'rational goal' (**Table 1**) [43, 49]:

- Human relations emphasizes flexibility and internal focus and stresses cohesion, human resource development and morale.
- Open relations emphasizes flexibility and external focus and stresses innovation, readiness and development.
- Internal process emphasizes control and internal focus and stresses stability, communication and control.
- Rational goal emphasizes control and external focus and stresses efficiency, goal setting and productivity.

All four culture types can be presented in a single organization, although some values are likely to be dominant [49]. However, emphasis on one organizational culture type can lead to narrowness and an inability to adapt to a changing environment [49]. When translating this to medical education, flexible medical schools (culture-type 'human relations' and/or 'open systems') tend to respond more positively to change than those featuring control-driven policies (culture-type 'rational goal' and/or 'internal process') [45]. A certain level of risk-taking, flexible policies, strong leadership, teamwork and strict hierarchy are some of the positive effects of organizational culture on curriculum change [45]. More specifically, risk-taking and flexible policies stimulated the introduction of innovative ideas and transdisciplinary teamwork is thought to be advantageous for integrated curricula, whereas strict hierarchy is believed to have a positive impact on the coordination of complex change [45].

3.4. Changing the behavior of medical doctors: a challenge in itself

So far, we have discussed the current use of change management in medical education, implementing change in complex systems and different contexts as well as the influence of culture on change. But what do we know about the adopters, that is, the trainees and medical specialists

	Internal	**External**
Flexibility	Human relations	Open systems
Control	Internal process	Rational goal

The competing values framework developed by Quinn et al. [49] explores competing demands within an organization on two axes. This leads to the four possible culture types, that is, 'human relations,' 'open systems,' 'internal process' and 'rational goal,' represented in this 2 × 2 table.

Table 1. Adapted from the competing values framework developed by Quinn et al. [49].

http://dx.doi.org/10.5772/intechopen.72113

confronted with curriculum change? Generally speaking, you could state that all organizational change starts with individual behavior change. Many theories of individual change have been published, but little research has been done to gain understanding of the dynamic interplay between individuals and the organization within which they work, and how the interplay influences individual or organizational behavior change [17]. Behavioral change is difficult, not only because it involves learning and implementing new knowledge but also, maybe even more important, it involves unlearning of old habits [50].

Lewin [2] states that behavior of individuals is the result of a balance between change drivers and restraining forces, leading to a quasi-stationary equilibrium (**Figure 2**) [2, 22]. Examples of change drivers are strong leadership, social demands or political forces, whereas examples of restraining forces are poor leadership, change fatigue or lack of time [2]. Lewin developed a linear three-stage model of change, starting with unfreezing of the status quo, followed by a change or transition leading to refreezing, that is, a new equilibrium. In the unfreezing phase, you need to create a state of 'readiness to change' in order to successfully start implementing the proposed change in the moving or transition phase. In the refreezing phase, the change must be adapted as the new way of practice and needs to sustain in order to create a new equilibrium [2]. In this model, change is seen as an isolated step in the process of transitioning from one stable equilibrium to the next. During this transition, efficiency or performance can decline due to, for instance, unfamiliarity with the new way of working or frustration as a result of that. Werther [51] calls this the learning curve of change (**Figure 2**). **Figure 2** combines the three-stage model of change of Lewin with the learning curve of Werther [22, 51].

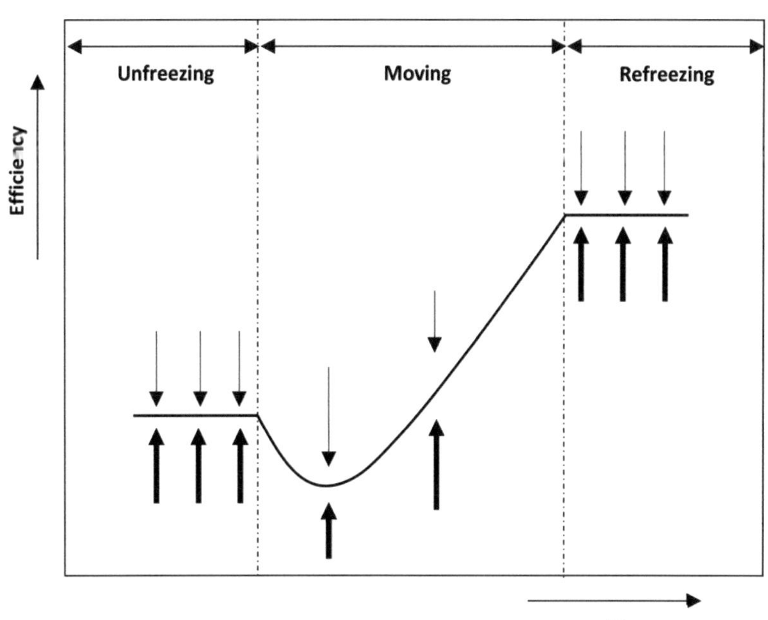

Figure 2. Three-stage model of change of Lewin. Three-stage model of change by Lewin [2], i.e. unfreezing, moving and refreezing. Thick black arrows facing upwards: change drivers. Thin black arrows facing downwards: restraining forces. The black line represents the learning curve of change by Werther and Davis [51].

However, the linear approach of Lewin seems not completely transferable to behavioral change in medical practice. Research has shown that medical doctors find it difficult to adopt new practices and have problems completely unlearning their old routines [50]. First, this might be due to the fact the many of the behaviors shown by medical doctors are deeply rooted habitual reflexes [52]. During their many years of training, starting at medical school, they have been exposed to countless guidelines or norms of practice behavior in both formal and informal ways. Moreover, repetitive assessment of these values, attitudes and skills by means of observation or drills are an integral part of their training. Together, this explains the strong anchoring of habits in medical doctors [52]. Second, medical doctors are generally highly ethical and professional and motivated by multiple interests such as their own interest, the patient's interest, and the interest of society. They must balance these with a professional ethos that demands, among other things, accountability and competence. As a result, the impact of change on clinical outcomes is important in the adoption of innovation [52]. Furthermore, the medical profession has a very prominent professional autonomy, and research in this field has shown that the profession tends to resist external pressures that either try to increase the control of medical practice [53] or try to influence the implementation processes [9, 19].

When confronted with practice change, medical doctors go through a process of trail-and-error while unlearning, developing their own method of implementation and building comfort with the new practice. Usually, they also develop personalized contingency theories based on patient characteristics that help them to decide in which case they should rely on the new practice rather than the old and vice versa [50]. For instance, medical doctors find it difficult to solely base their practice change on literature and rely on discussion with their colleagues on how to incorporate new guidelines into daily practice [50]. Additionally, the quality of evidence behind the new guidelines is an important factor in determining whether medical doctors will use this evidence to support their unlearning. So, in practice, the unlearning process of medical doctors is less fluent as might be suggested by the linear model of Lewin. Already mentioned earlier, medical innovations tend to be added to the already existing repertoire of diagnostic or therapeutic options rather than replacing them [24]. Additionally, the adaption of new practice introduces further change as medical doctors are discussing, self-reflecting and evaluating the new practice with their colleagues. You could say that the medical profession is in a continuous stage of change [6, 50].

4. Readiness for change

In such a dynamic and constantly changing environment, it is important to know whether the people involved are psychologically and behaviorally prepared to implement the proposed change [54]. Therefore, one of the potentially beneficial change management strategies for PGME could be the assessment of organizational readiness for change (ORC) [9]. Organizational readiness for change reflects the degree to which members of an organization are collectively primed, motivated and capable to adopt and execute a particular change initiative to purposefully alter the status quo [55]. It is believed that organizational readiness for change is a critical precursor for successful implementation of complex change initiatives in healthcare settings

[21, 54]. When change leaders establish insufficient readiness, a range of predictable and undesirable outcomes could occur: change efforts make a false start from which it might or might not recover, change efforts stall as resistance grows, or the change fails altogether [54].

Change readiness is a comprehensive, multifaceted construct as it comprises both psychological and structural factors that together determine the degree of readiness present [54, 55]. Psychological factors reflect the extent to which the members of the organization are cognitively and emotionally inclined to implement the proposed change [55]. For instance, 'collective efficacy' reflects the shared belief in a team's conjoint capabilities to organize and execute the right actions to successfully implement change, whereas 'appropriateness' reflects the belief a change is correct for the situation being addressed [55]. These beliefs relate to the amount of effort that team members are willing to put into a change process, that is, when change seems unreachable, possible obstacles seem harder to encounter and change efforts are low [4, 56]. Structural factors reflect the extent to which the circumstances under which the change is occurring enhance or inhibit the implementation of the proposed change [55]. Examples are whether or not a team's skills and abilities align with the actions that need to be taken and the presence of both a tangible environment (e.g., funding) and an intangible environment (e.g., culture) to support change [55]. When looking at organizational readiness, it is important to stress the collective nature of this construct. Implementing complex change initiatives in healthcare settings requires collective action of those involved, each of whom contributes their share to the implementation process [54]. When ORC is high, the staff involved are more dedicated to contribute to the proposed change process and more persistent in the event of setbacks. Conversely, when ORC is low, the staff involved are more likely to consider change as undesirable and may avoid or even resist participation [4, 54, 55, 57, 58]. Team members will commit to a change because they either want to, have to or ought to. Regardless of its reason, this form of commitment will lead to behavioral compliance. Some, however, might show resistance, either active or passive, and fail to comply [59]. Actions to create readiness include among others establishing a sense of urgency, empowering your team members and creating an appealing vision for the future as well as fostering a sense of confidence that this can be realized [9, 21, 54]. Change readiness can be assessed at several stages of the change process, that is, before or during change, as a way to diagnose any possible or current hurdles in the implementation process in order to facilitate any corrective interventions. Additionally, readiness can be assessed repeatedly to explore the effects of these interventions [9].

4.1. Readiness for change in postgraduate medical education

In the last decade, the attention for ORC increased, leading to the development of multiple instruments to assess ORC in healthcare. Generally, these instruments tend to focus on the implementation of new guidelines or new practices [57, 60]. In undergraduate medical education, several instruments were developed as well [9, 61, 62]. However, in postgraduate medical education, only one instrument to assess ORC exists, that is, Specialty Training's Organizational Readiness for curriculum Change (STORC) [9]. STORC was designed to measure readiness for change in clinical teaching teams, that is, a hospital-based educational team within one department, such as radiology or gynecology, consisting of a program director, clinical staff members and trainees. STORC was developed specifically for this setting as it was expected that the use of the former instruments would not take into account the unique properties of PGME [9]. In teaching hospitals, PGME is completely integrated into clinical service, that is, patient care, teaching and learning are interconnected to each other and cannot be seen separately [63]. Therefore, any adjustments made to the educational system will influence clinical service and could have consequences for, e.g., working schedules, funding and learning experiences [9, 63]. Furthermore, instruments developed for undergraduate medical education focus on medical faculties, to the neglect of students, with long-lasting hierarchical structures, leading to a more diverse set of pressures to change [9, 61]. Additionally, trainees have a far more active role in implementing curricula than medical students [14, 64] and work in smaller clinical teaching teams that tend to have a more volatile composition than medical faculties [9].

Through an international Delphi procedure, the applicability of a questionnaire to assess ORC in PGME was determined. The preliminary questionnaire was based on existing instruments derived from business and healthcare settings [9]. In two Delphi rounds, the 41 expert panelists (trainees and medical specialists from four different countries) determined the most important and applicable items and subscales to assess ORC in PGME. This Delphi procedure was followed by confirmatory factor analysis validating the clustering of items within the 10 subscales (**Table 2**) [19].

The final subscale consists out of 43 items divided into 10 subscales [19]. Together, they represent both psychological and structural factors as well as most of the core components of ORC

Subscales STORC [9, 19]	Topic(s) covered
Pressure to change	Which sources exert pressure to implement a particular change in residency training and to what extent?
Appropriateness	Is the innovation in residency training appropriate for the situation being addressed?
Necessity to change	Is there a significant difference between the current state and the desired state of residency training?
Management support and leadership	Is the educational board (hospital level) committed to and support the change initiative?
Staff culture	Do clinical staff members cooperate and share responsibilities and are they willing to innovate?
The formal leader	Does the program director accept responsibility and have the authority to lead the implementation of a particular change?
Involvement	How is the quality of change communication?
Project resources	Which recourses are available to implement a particular change in residency training and to what extent?
Clarity of mission and goals	Are team members aware of the mission and goals of the change?
The implementation plan	Is there an implementation plan that among others describes tasks, timelines and an evaluation plan?

Subscales and topics covered by the questionnaire specialty training's organizational readiness for curriculum change (STORC). The questionnaire covers all core components of organizational readiness for change described in literature [9, 19].

Table 2. Subscales and topics covered by the questionnaire STORC (adapted from Bank [16]).

described in literature (**Table 2**) [9, 19]. Since ORC is measured on various subscales and presented as such, its strength lies in analyzing these subscales. The latter makes it possible for educational leaders to identify and anticipate on hurdles in the implementation process at an early stage, or more ideally, prior to change. Subsequently, change efforts could be optimized by targeted interventions aimed at facilitating successful curriculum change. The effect of these interventions could be measured by repeated administration of STORC [9].

During the development of STORC [9, 19], it became apparent that external pressures, such as hospital boards accreditation bodies and the ministry of health were not represented in the final version of STORC despite the fact that CBME is top-down driven [9, 19]. Possibly, external pressures are not experienced on a daily basis, explaining the exclusion of these pressures in STORC. Alternatively, hospitals are not organized according to the habitual management practices, leading to a different set of (recognized) pressures [19, 65]. Alternatively, as mentioned earlier, medical doctors have a very prominent professional autonomy which might make them less receptive to external pressure [19].

After its development, STORC was used to assess ORC in PGME in the Netherlands, in order to understand how clinical teaching teams deal with curriculum change such as the introduction of CBME. The level of ORC is measured at the individual level but aggregated to team levels in the analysis. By looking at the team's 'state' of readiness for change, insights were gathered regarding leadership roles, teamwork, shared commitment, perceived support and behavioral reactions to change [16].

When comparing the different subscales of STORC, one important trend can be seen (**Table 3**). The subscale 'formal leader,' consisting of items regarding whether the program director has the authority to lead and accepts responsibility for the success of the change process, scored higher than the other scales. High scores were also given on the subscale 'staff culture,' which includes items about teamwork and clinical staff's receptiveness to changes, as well as on the subscale 'appropriateness.' At the other end, the subscales 'management support and leadership,' 'project recourses' and 'implementation plan' had the lowest scores [16].

These results clearly designate the program director as the leader of educational change. This is in line with change literature that shows implementation is accelerated in the presence of leaders that function as role models and entrepreneurs [14]. Strong leadership will also help clinical team members to adjust habits and routines [15]. High scores on the subscale 'staff culture' show that clinical staff members do feel and share a sense of responsibility for the

Highest scoring subscales of STORC	Lowest scoring subscales of STORC
Formal leader	Management support and leadership
Staff culture	Implementation plan
Appropriateness	Project resources

Results of the assessment of readiness for change in clinical teaching teams in the Netherlands. The table shows the subscales of STORC that had the highest and lowest scores throughout the sample of respondents, that is, program directors, clinical staff members and trainees.

Table 3. Subscales of questionnaire STORC showing the highest and lowest scores [16].

improvement of training which is in line with the philosophy of CBME [40]. High scores on the subscale 'appropriateness' suggest CBME indeed seems to meet the needs in PGME and is therefore accepted as an appropriate innovation [16].

The lowest scores were seen on the subscales 'management support and leadership,' 'project recourses' and 'implementation plan,' all representing components related to change management. In the light of the limited attention to change management principles in medical education, this was not surprising and puts emphasis on the absence of descriptions of tasks and timelines, and the shortage of evaluation cycles, training facilities and financial resources [16].

In sum, clinical teaching teams appear to comply with the implementation of curriculum change if the proposed change is seen as a correct innovation. In that case, program directors receive and take the responsibility for the job that needs to be done, but they lack a fully equipped toolbox of change management principles to actually implement change as efficiently as possible [16].

5. Practical implications

To come back to the adopter categories of Rogers [18], many would expect that you should focus on targeting the late majority and laggards to speed up diffusion of innovation. However, they are also the hardest to convince and will probably not even consider changing until the idea has become well accepted by a solid majority of the target audience. It is much easier to reach and convince innovators or early adopters. Rogers calls them the 'critical mass.' Once 15% of the population has adopted a new idea, it has the critical mass to spread on its own momentum. This is named the tipping point. Furthermore, people in these categories are considered to be leaders and are well respected, so their peers will be more likely to pick up the new behavior [18].

Looking at the literature on how medical doctors deal with practice change gives valuable insights on how to introduce educational change as well. Medical doctors tend to discuss the information presented to them among each other and subsequently translate this into their own practice. Furthermore, they weigh the evidence and consequences for patient outcomes [50]. This particular process of translating theory into practice by solely the profession itself underscores the professional autonomy a medical doctor has. When correlating this to the diffusion of innovation theory of Rogers [18] and the five innovation attributes he describes, the trialability of an educational innovation is particularly important to consider. Trialability implies a certain degree of freedom to experiment with the innovation when implementing it, which clearly relates to the professional autonomy medical doctors experience when implementing clinical practice change. That said, trialability might also lead to a certain degree of reinvention if allowed without a purposeful amount of structure. Reinvention could be valuable to simplify a complex innovation to a local context. However, it could also result in suboptimal implementation of change such as we have seen with the implementation of the seven roles of CanMEDS. The abstract description of these roles led to a lack of clarity about their content, meaning and relevance in clinical practice [5, 30, 31, 66]. Subsequently, adequate implementation was hampered [14, 25].

There is no single solution which will trigger or ensure adequate educational innovation, as the interaction between the innovation and the context of its introduction is necessarily complex and variable [3]. Achieving a sufficient level of ORC in itself does not guarantee the implementation of a complex change will result in the anticipated success [54]. Therefore, a multifaceted approach is essential such as combining the assessment of ORC prior to change [9, 19], with ensuring adequate innovation attributes [18] and being receptive to the specific characteristics of behavioral change by medical doctors [9, 19, 50].

6. Conclusion

Attention to change management support in postgraduate medical education is a change for the better. It could help guide implementation processes, optimize change efforts, avoid the use of ineffective strategies, save time and money, prolong sustainability of change and potentially promote the dissemination of findings in other contexts. However, a 'one size fits all' approach probably does not work as the interaction between the innovation and the organizational context, including the influence of culture, can vary. Therefore, a multifaceted approach is advised combining multiple change management principles as well as insight from behavioral change in medical practice. As educational objectives continue to change and curriculum standards continue to evolve, change is a continuous process that requires the people involved to learn to change and to change to learn.

Abbreviations

CBME	Competency based medical education.
PGME	Postgraduate medical education.
STORC	Specialty Trainings' Organizational Readiness for curriculum Change.
ORC	Organizational readiness for change.
EPA	Entrustable professional activity.
STAR	Statement of awarded responsibility.
ACGME	Accreditation Council of Graduate Medical Education.

Author details

Lindsay Bank[1]*, Mariëlle Jippes[2], Albert J.J.A. Scherpbier[3] and Fedde Scheele[1,4,5,6]

*Address all correspondence to: bank.lindsay@gmail.com

1 Department of Healthcare Education, OLVG Hospital, Amsterdam, The Netherlands

2 Department of Plastic Surgery, Erasmus Medical Centre, Rotterdam, The Netherlands

3 Institute of Medical Education, Faculty of Health, Medicine and Life Sciences, Maastricht University, Maastricht, The Netherlands

4 Athena Institute for Trans Disciplinary Research, Vu University, Amsterdam, The Netherlands

5 Medical School of Sciences, Vu University Medical Centre, Amsterdam, The Netherlands

6 Department of Gynaecology, OLVG Hospital, Amsterdam, The Netherlands

References

[1] London M. The Oxford Handbook of Lifelong Learning. Oxford University Press; New York, USA. 2011

[2] Lewin K, Lewin GW. Resolving Social Conflicts: Selected Papers on Group Dynamics. New York, NY: Harper & Row; 1948

[3] Williams I. Organizational readiness for innovation in health care: Some lessons from the recent literature. Health Services Management Research. 2011;**24**:213-218

[4] Weiner BJ, Amick H, Lee SY. Conceptualization and measurement of organizational readiness for change: A review of the literature in health services research and other fields. Medical Care Research and Review. 2008;**65**:379-436

[5] Scheele F, Van Luijk S, Mulder H, Baane C, den Rooyen C, de Hoog M, et al. Is the modernisation of postgraduate medical training in the Netherlands successful? Views of the NVMO special interest group on postgraduate medical education. Medical Teacher. 2014;**36**:116-120

[6] Schultz K, Griffiths J. Implementing competency-based medical education in a postgraduate family medicine residency training program: A stepwise approach, facilitating factors, and processes or steps that would have been helpful. Academic Medicine. 2016;**91**:685-689

[7] Frank JR, Snell L, Sherbino J, editors. CanMEDS 2015 Physician Competency Framework. Royal College of Physicians and Surgeons of Canada: Ottawa; 2015

[8] Carraccio C, Englander R, Van Melle E, ten Cate O, Lockyer J, Chan MK, et al. Advancing competency-based medical education: A charter for clinician-educators. Academic Medicine. 2015

[9] Bank L, Jippes M, Van Luijk S, den Rooyen C, Scherpbier A, Scheele F. Specialty Training's Organizational Readiness for curriculum Change (STORC): Development of a questionnaire in a Delphi study. BMC Medical Education. 2015;**15**:127

[10] Consoli D, Mina A. An evolutionary perspective on health innovations systems. Journal of Evolutionary Economics. 2009;**19**:297-319

[11] Harlos K, Tetroe J, Graham ID, Bird M, Robinson N. Mining the management literature for insights into implementing evidence-based change in healthcare. Healthc Policy. 2012; **8**:33-48

[12] Ferlie E, Fitzgerald L, Wood M, Hawkins C. The nonspread of innovations: The mediating role of professionals. The Academy of Management Journal. 2005;**48**:117-134

[13] Fleuren M, Wiefferink K, Paulussen T. Determinants of innovation within health care organizations: Literature review and Delphi study. International Journal for Quality in Health Care. 2004;**16**:107-123

[14] Jippes E, Van Luijk SJ, Pols J, Achterkamp MC, Brand PL, van Engelen JM. Facilitators and barriers to a nationwide implementation of competency-based postgraduate medical curricula: A qualitative study. Medical Teacher. 2012;**34**:e589-e602

[15] Greenhalgh T, Robert G, Macfarlane F, Bate P, Kyriakidou O. Diffusion of innovations in service organizations: Systematic review and recommendations. The Milbank Quarterly. 2004;**82**:581-629

[16] Bank L, Jippes M, Leppink J, Scherpbier AJ, den Rooyen C, van Luijk SJ, Scheele F. Are they ready? Organizational readiness for change among clinical teaching teams. Advances in Medical Education and Practice. 2017;**8**:807-815

[17] Damschroder LJ, Aron DC, Keith RE, Kirsh SR, Alexander JA, Lowery JC. Fostering implementation of health services research findings into practice: A consolidated framework for advancing implementation science. Implementation Science. 2009;**4**:50

[18] Rogers EM. Diffusion of Innovations. 5th ed. New York: Free Press; 2005

[19] Bank L, Jippes M, Leppink J, Scherpbier AJ, den Rooyen C, van Luijk SJ, Scheele F. Specialty Training's Organizational Readiness for curriculum Change (STORC): Validation of a questionnaire. Advances in Medical Education and Practice. 2018;**9**:75-83

[20] Rafferty AE, Jimmieson NL, Armenakis AA. Change readiness: A multilevel review. Journal of Management. 2013;**39**:110-135

[21] Kotter JP. Leading Change. Boston, MA: Harvard Business School Press; 1996

[22] Cozijnsen AJ, Vrakking WJ. Handbook Change Management. [Dutch] Deventer: Vakmedianet; 2015

[23] Carlfjord S, Lindberg M, Bendtsen P, Nilsen P, Andersson A. Key factors influencing adoption of an innovation in primary health care: A qualitative study based on implementation theory. BMC Family Practice. 2010;**11**:60

[24] Djellal F, Gallouj F. Innovation in hospital: A survey of the literature. The European Journal of Health Economics. 2007;**8**:181-193

[25] Lillevang G, Bugge L, Beck H, Joost-Rethans J, Ringsted C. Evaluation of a national process of reforming curricula in postgraduate medical education. Medical Teacher. 2009;**31**:e260-e266

[26] Frank JR, Danoff D. The CanMEDS initiative: Implementing an outcomes-based framework of physician competencies. Medical Teacher. 2007;**29**:642-647

[27] Scheele F, Teunissen P, Van Luijk S, Heineman E, Fluit L, Mulder H, et al. Introducing competency-based postgraduate medical education in the Netherlands. Medical Teacher. 2008;**30**:248-253

[28] ten Cate O, Scheele F. Competency-based postgraduate training: Can we bridge the gap between theory and clinical practice? Academic Medicine. 2007;**82**:542-547

[29] McEwen LA, Griffiths J, Schultz K. Developing and successfully implementing a competency-based portfolio assessment system in a postgraduate family medicine residency program. Academic Medicine. 2015;**90**:1515-1526

[30] Chou S, Cole G, McLaughlin K, Lockyer J. CanMEDS evaluation in Canadian postgraduate training programmes: Tools used and programme director satisfaction. Medical Education. 2008;**42**:879-886

[31] Ringsted C, Hansen TL, Davis D, Scherpbier A. Are some of the challenging aspects of the CanMEDS roles valid outside Canada? Medical Education. 2006;**40**:807-815

[32] Hawkins RE, Welcher CM, Holmboe ES, Kirk LM, Norcini JJ, Simons KB, et al. Implementation of competency-based medical education: Are we addressing the concerns and challenges? Medical Education. 2015;**49**:1086-1102

[33] Plsek PE, Greenhalgh T. Complexity science: The challenge of complexity in health care. British Medical Journal. 2001;**323**:625-628

[34] van Rossum TR, Scheele F, Scherpbier AJ, Sluiter HE, Heyligers IC. Dealing with the complex dynamics of teaching hospitals. BMC Medical Education. 2016;**16**:104

[35] Plsek PE, Wilson T. Complexity, leadership, and management in healthcare organisations. British Medical Journal. 2001;**323**:746-749

[36] Lowenstein SR, Fernandez G, Crane LA. Medical school faculty discontent: Prevalence and predictors of intent to leave academic careers. BMC Medical Education. 2007;**7**:37

[37] Fairchild DG, Benjamin EM, Gifford DR, Huot SJ. Physician leadership: Enhancing the career development of academic physician administrators and leaders. Academic Medicine. 2004;**79**:214-218

[38] Beasley BW, Simon SD, Wright SM. A time to be promoted. The prospective study of promotion in academia (prospective study of promotion in academia). Journal of General Internal Medicine. 2006;**21**:123-129

[39] Pololi L, Kern DE, Carr P, Conrad P, Knight S. The culture of academic medicine: Faculty perceptions of the lack of alignment between individual and institutional values. Journal of General Internal Medicine. 2009;**24**:1289-1295

[40] Frank JR. Royal College of Physicians and Surgeons of Canada: The CanMEDS 2005 Physician Competency Framework: Better Standards, Better Physicians, Better Care. Royal College of Physicians and Surgeons of Canada: Ottawa, Ontario; 2005

[41] ACGME Common Program Requirements. Accreditation Council for Graduate Medical Education. Jun 9, 2013. Available from: http://www.acgme.org/acgmeweb/Portals/0/PFAssets/ProgramRequirements/CPRs2013.pdf

[42] van der Aa JE, Tancredi A, Goverde AJ, Velebil P, Feyereisl J, Benedetto C, et al. What European gynaecologists need to master: Consensus on medical expertise outcomes of pan-European postgraduate training in obstetrics & gynaecology. European Journal of Obstetrics, Gynecology, and Reproductive Biology. 2017;**216**:143-152

[43] Jones RA, Jimmieson NL, Griffiths A. The impact of organizational culture and reshaping capabilities on change implementation success: The mediating role of readiness for change. Journal of Management Studies. 2005;**42**:361-386

[44] Ingersoll GL, Kirsch JC, Merk SE, Lightfoot J. Relationship of organizational culture and readiness for change to employee commitment to the organization. The Journal of Nursing Administration. 2000;**30**:11-20

[45] Jippes M, Driessen EW, Broers NJ, Majoor GD, Gijselaers WH, van der Vleuten CP. Culture matters in successful curriculum change: An international study of the influence of national and organizational culture tested with multilevel structural equation Modeling. Academic Medicine. 2015;**90**:921-929

[46] Jippes M, Majoor GD. Influence of national culture on the adoption of integrated medical curricula. Advances in Health Sciences Education: Theory and Practice. 2011;**16**:5-16

[47] Cook N, Yanow D. Culture and organizational learning. Journal of Management Inquiry. 2011;**20**:362-379

[48] Schein EH: Organizational Culture and Leadership: [A Dynamic View]. San Francisco, Calif: Jossey-Bass, 1985

[49] Quinn RE, Hildebrandt HW, Rogers PS, Thompson MP. A competing values framework for analyzing presentational communication in management contexts. Journal of Business Communication. 1991;**28**:213-232

[50] Gupta DM, Boland RJ Jr, Aron DC. The physician's experience of changing clinical practice: A struggle to unlearn. Implementation Science. 2017;**12**:28

[51] Werther WB. Human Resources and Personnel Management. 5th ed. New York: Mc Graw Hill; 1996

[52] Smith WR. Evidence for the effectiveness of techniques to change physician behavior. Chest. 2000;**118**:8S-17S

[53] Kitchener M. The 'Bureaucratization' of professional roles: The case of clinical directors in UK hospitals. Organization. 2000;**7**:129-154

[54] Weiner BJ. A theory of organizational readiness for change. Implementation Science. 2009;**4**:67

[55] Holt DT, Helfrich CD, Hall CG, Weiner BJ. Are you ready? How health professionals can comprehensively conceptualize readiness for change. Journal of General Internal Medicine. 2010;**25**:50-55

[56] Holt D, Armenakis A, Feild H, Harris S. Readiness for organizational change: The systematic development of scale. The Journal of Applied Behavioral Science. 2007;**43**:232-255

[57] Shea CM, Jacobs SR, Esserman DA, Bruce K, Weiner BJ. Organizational readiness for implementing change: A psychometric assessment of a new measure. Implementation Science. 2014;**9**:7

[58] Lehman WE, Greener JM, Simpson DD. Assessing organizational readiness for change. Journal of Substance Abuse Treatment. 2002;**22**:197-209

[59] Herscovitch L, Meyer JP. Commitment to organizational change: Extension of a three-component model. The Journal of Applied Psychology. 2002;**87**:474-487

[60] Helfrich CD, Li YF, Sharp ND, Sales AE. Organizational readiness to change assessment (ORCA): Development of an instrument based on the promoting action on research in health services (PARIHS) framework. Implementation Science. 2009;**4**:38

[61] Jippes M, Driessen EW, Broers NJ, Majoor GD, Gijselaers WH, van der Vleuten CP. A medical school's organizational readiness for curriculum change (MORC): Development and validation of a questionnaire. Academic Medicine. 2013;**88**:1346-1356

[62] Malau-Aduli BS, Zimitat C, Malau-Aduli AEO. Quality assured assessment processes evaluating staff response to change. Higher Education Management and Policy. 2011; **23**:1-24

[63] Billett S. Constituting the workplace curriculum. Journal of Curriculum Studies. 2006; **38**:31-48

[64] Jippes E, van Engelen JM, Brand PL, Oudkerk M. Competency-based (CanMEDS) residency training programme in radiology: Systematic design procedure, curriculum and success factors. European Radiology. 2010;**20**:967-977

[65] Witman Y, Smid GAC, Meurs PL, Willems DL. Doctor in the lead: Balancing between two worlds. Organization. 2011;**18**:477-495

[66] Zibrowski EM, Singh SI, Goldszmidt MA, Watling CJ, Kenyon CF, Schulz V, et al. The sum of the parts detracts from the intended whole: Competencies and in-training assessments. Medical Education. 2009;**43**:741-748

Chapter 4

Role of Protected Block Curriculum in Surgical Education

Philip N. Redlich, Travis P. Webb and
John A. Weigelt

Additional information is available at the end of the chapter

http://dx.doi.org/10.5772/intechopen.72120

Abstract

A protected block curriculum for surgical resident training began at the Medical College of Wisconsin in 2005. The curriculum has evolved with time as educational emphasis has changed. However, the concept of having resident learners relieved of clinical duty to focus on learning has not changed. Separate protected block curriculums are held for PGY1 and PGY 2 during which residents have no clinical responsibilities. These periods are defined at the beginning of each academic year and are distributed to all faculties. The systematic design, implementation, and evaluation of the protected block curriculum (PBC) Model provides an educationally grounded model for training surgical residents consistent with accreditation council for graduate medical education (ACGME) competency mandates. Resident evaluations consistently support the use of our PBC as a method to attain and practice skill sets in a nonthreatening environment. Faculty benefits are able to evaluate residents' knowledge, skills, and attitudes in a nonclinical setting and engage residents as individuals. The format extended into the PGY3–5 years of training as it evolved. Over more than a decade of using PBC, we have performed a number of analyses on the program and even determined a cost for the program. The program continues to be adjusted to new technology and curriculum initiatives.

Keywords: surgical education, protected block curriculum

1. Introduction

The general surgery residency educational mission at the Medical College of Wisconsin (MCW) was under scrutiny in the beginning of the year 2002. Many key stakeholders voiced concerns that residents were not receiving the optimal educational experience preparing them for the continuum of residency and future clinical practice. A number of options to address perceived educational shortcomings were presented to the department, but given interim leadership in the office of Chairman, no decision endorsing significant change was considered until 2004. In late 2004, department leadership stabilized and agreed that many of our PGY1 residents were struggling with the challenges in their first year of training, especially in the early months of their PGY1 year. Numerous reasons were offered and debated for this problem, but an obvious solution was the restructuring of the initial PGY 1 year of resident training. At the time, very little structured curriculum existed specifically for the PGY1 residents outside service or department wide major conferences such as weekly grand rounds and morbidity and mortality (M&M) conference. A weekly lecture series for residents existed, but topics were targeted to the upper-level residents. Each service had defined objectives that were specific for the service based on the patient populations served, but there was a lack of standardization of how those specific objectives were taught and assessed. The ACGME competencies had been recently introduced and numerous domains of the program were not specifically addressed by the current residency curriculum.

In response to this realization, the Program Director and the Chair of Surgery agreed to evaluate the current curriculum and plan a new curriculum for the next academic year. A scholarly approach to the change was taken by following Kotter's eight-step process of change as a scaffolding for improving the educational program [1]. The process started with a planning committee composed of a small group of key faculty and residents who met and discussed the strengths and weaknesses of our current curriculum. These meetings were facilitated by a PhD educator from the Division of Educational Services in the Office of Academic Affairs at MCW. The matrix for these sessions used six domains of the ACGME Competency Program: medical knowledge, patient care, professionalism, interpersonal and communication skills, practice-based learning and improvement (PBL&I), and systems-based practice (SBP). A list of topics in each area was developed based on the current literature and our existing curricular objectives, since there was no available guidance on topics from surgical associations or organizations [2–5]. Additionally, a number of models were developed for the implementation of a new curriculum. The assumptions used to create these models are outlined in **Table 1**.

Two meetings were planned as retreats for the faculty including faculty from affiliate teaching sites and resident representatives. The first meeting highlighted the changes occurring

1. Compliant with the 80h work.
2. Encourage an environment that is conducive to learning.
3. Continue to expect residents to attend our major teaching conferences during this learning period (Grand rounds and M&M).
4. Core services will have at least three residents.
5. Proposed curriculum identified 240 h contact time for the first 3 years of residency. PGY1 time was 52 didactic hours, 48 case scenario discussions, 92 h of simulation, 24 h of the literature review, and 24 h of communication skills.
6. The learning day could be 6 or 8 h long.

Table 1. Assumptions used to construct models.

in surgical education and the direction that the ACGME and Residency Review Committees (RRC) were taking. The urgency to respond to these changes was clearly delineated. The next step involved a presentation of the topics and the planning committee felt that it was necessary to cover in each of the ACGME competency domains. It was clear that the list was very long, and one of the tasks of this first retreat was to prioritize the topics for the PGY1 residents. This task was accomplished by splitting the faculty attendees into three groups and asking for their review. The final step of this first meeting was to present four models proposed by the planning committee. A small amount of discussion occurred to explain the rationale for the models. The action item for the participants was to review the material from the retreat and come prepared for the next meeting to make decisions about the curriculum model, we would implement.

Two weeks later, the second meeting was held. Two objectives were planned: (1) a review of curriculum topics and (2) decision on the model that we would use for the curriculum. A small number of changes were made in the topic list. Some specific additions included items for professionalism and communication especially with allied healthcare professionals. The major discussion was on the model that would be used as the chosen model since it would have the greatest impact on all stakeholders. A principle that was adopted, though with some hesitation, was that time for the curriculum must be free of clinical duties including overnight call responsibilities starting around noon on Saturday, the weekend prior to the curriculum. This item was the major change debated. A significant concern was the ability to support operative cases whether the PGY1 residents were not on clinical duty. Facilitators continued to keep the educational mission at the forefront and a final decision supporting the need to have protected time for educational activities won the discussion. The four models discussed are briefly outlined in **Table 2**.

A model E was brought forward from the participants. This model had a concentrated time period before the PGY1 residents actually started on clinical service followed by intermittent regular sessions. After considering the logistics of this model, it was also declined.

The final decision was to use model B. The PGY1 residents were informed of the curriculum the last week of June as their orientation sessions were held. This end-of-June session would extend a few days into July as an introduction to the overall curriculum. The actual "first semester" would be a week in August, September, and October. We would take a winter break in November and December. The "second semester" would be a week in January, February, March, and April. Graduation week in May would only be a couple of days.

Model A	2 days/week (with day off preceding to stay compliant with duty hours)	Declined
Model B	1 week–5.5 days/month	Accepted
Model C	2 weeks quarterly	Declined
Model D	Entire block of time 1 month	Declined

Table 2. The various types of curriculum models discussed during the faculty retreats.

The entire faculty agreed that our new protected block curriculum (PBC) would be free from service and on-call responsibilities, a week in duration, and continuous throughout the year. The schedule called for sessions Monday through Friday morning, with time used on Sunday for the completion of required materials including homework.

2. Maturation of the protected block curriculum

2.1. First year

Planning for the first year of our PBC began immediately. Faculty volunteers (champions) for the various aspects of the curriculum were recruited, and assignments were made for the entire year. Each session was planned to cover essentials for our PGY1 curriculum (**Table 3** attached). The faculty were divided into teams based on their topic assignments. An example of the competency domains and team leaders for our first week of the PBC are shown in **Table 4**.

Each month's curriculum was developed and teaching sessions were assigned to instructors. The majority of teaching was assigned to the surgical faculty, although we benefited from the expertise of several other departments when relevant. Sessions covering imaging were given by our colleagues from the Department of Radiology.

Cardiac complications were covered by cardiologists. Educators from our Department of Education helped with communication topics. Novel approaches to education such as videotaping resident presentations were used to help residents to review their communication skills. Medical knowledge was assessed at the conclusion of each block by using preexams and postexams covering material taught in each session. Skills assessments were performed for skill stations by using defined objectives for performance. Each session was evaluated by our residents and their comments were used to make changes in topics covered, presenters within or outside the Department, time spent on each topic, and decisions on future topics for upcoming months as well as future years [6].

A unique aspect of the PBC was the addition of the surgical learning and instructional portfolio (SLIP). [7]. This educational resource was developed based on recommendations from the ACGME toolbox. The residents were asked to identify a case that they encountered each month. They were required to describe a case history, review the diagnostic studies used, and present the differential diagnosis. A list of ICD9 codes and CPT codes was also required. Finally, a discussion of the case and lessons learned was required. These cases were reviewed by a faculty member and feedback provided. This activity was transitioned to all residents in 2010.

To administratively support the new PBC, a Division of Education within the Department of Surgery was established with a Chief, administrator, and administrative assistant that were important for the organizational success of the curriculum. This occurred in 2005. A Director of the PGY1 curriculum was designated.

The entire program was a resounding success. Feedback from our PGY1 residents was excellent. Feedback from our faculty was positive and surprising, as many faculty stated that they felt the

ACGME competencies	PGY 1[1]	PGY 2	PGY 3	PGY 4	PGY 5
Medical Knowledge					
Assessment of basic diagnostic tests	How tests are ordered at each institution, normal values, usefulness, which are helpful in clinical situations.				
Imaging	Chest radiograph and others consistent with scope of practice for year of training				
Instruments *Match K&S to Scope of practice by year*	Needed instruments for operations within the training year's expectations				
Nutrition					
Fluid and electrolytes	Commonly seen in surgical patients, core chapters in any text	Abdominal CT	Special abdominal CT exams		
Acid/base balance	Commonly seen in surgical patients				
Shock resuscitation	All four types				
Surgical infections	Surgical ID content				
Transfusion medicine	Use of blood components, basic coagulation information				
Pharmacokinetics	What is this, how can it help, how are drugs handled by metabolic pathways, common problems, use of PharmD colleagues in practice				
Endocrine	Diabetes in surgical patients, metabolism in surgical patients, catabolism, anabolism, use basic chapter information				
Patient care					
General	ACS-Ultrasound 101, ATLS ACLS if not already done this	US certification			

ACGME competencies	PGY 1[1]	PGY 2	PGY 3	PGY 4	PGY 5
Order writing	How to write admission orders, post-op orders for scope of practice, different orders at different hospitals, different computer systems				
Pre-op Assessments	Knowledge of pre-op test needs for general and regional anesthesia				
	Proper H and P for surgical procedure				
Use of consultants[2]	How to contact consultants	When to contact and how to ask the right question			
Out vs in-patient procedures	Appropriateness of site of procedure for outpatient and inpatient surgery, different systems for procedures within the program.				
Perioperative Management	Pre-op bowel preparation				
	Coagulation monitoring				
	Pre-op risk assessment, cardiac, pulmonary, infection, DVT, comorbidities,	Use of consultants			
	Management of drugs pre-op including dosing and holding during perioperative period				
	Know appropriate DVT protocols, Understand the risk analysis for DVT				
	Principles of perioperative antimicrobial prophylaxis				
	Stoma marking knowledge	Planning			

ACGME competencies	PGY 1[1]	PGY 2	PGY 3	PGY 4	PGY 5
	Reduction of surgical risk, maneuvers.				
	Draping, sterile field Basic tray and function OR Environment	Getting patient ready for appropriate procedure at skill level			
Operative skills, skill lab to achieve most of this as well as in the operating room	25% effort				
	Climate control in OR, proper patient position for the scope of practice Problem solving when possible Proper use of Bovie	Knowledge of lights, backup systems, lasers, CUSA			
	Roles and responsibilities of surgeon and assistant Skin preps Time management in OR OR Costs Instruments needed for various procedures again within scope of practice				
	Knots 1+ 2 handed	Stapling techniques Sewing Bowel Intro Lap Intra-op US	Knots and sutures x # /time period (efficiency) Wet labs in trauma surgery, general surgery, vascular surgery, minimally invasive surgery	Thoracic procedures	
	Management of various types of drains and tubes	Drains and tubes			
	Instruments and handling within scope of practice				
	Sutures				
	Materials and dressings such as VAC pack for abdominal closure, retention sutures, other wound dressings				

ACGME competencies	PGY 1[1]	PGY 2	PGY 3	PGY 4	PGY 5
	Amputation - Digit - Transmetatarsal - Above knee - Below knee - Digital Appendectomy Breast biopsy Bronchoscopy Circumcision Pilonidal Cyst drainage and removal Drain abscess -perirectal -Sub cutaneous Excision of: -Lymphoma -Skin lesion -Sub cutaneous lesions Hemorrhoidectomy Flexible sigmoidoscopy Gastrostomy Adult Hernia repair: - Ventral - Inguinal Hernia Pediatric Hernia Repair -Inguinal -Umbilical Hemorrhoidectomy Jejunostomy Major Wounds: -Suture -Debridement Remove: Skin moles -Small tumors -Subcutaneous cysts -Foreign bodies -Tumors	Cholecystectomy Small bowel resection Splenectomy Endoscopy upper and lower Central Venous: -Line placement -Percutaneous CV access -Implantation CV access devices Insertion: -Hickman catheters and other indwell catheters	Colectomy Advanced laparoscopic procedures Captain on trauma resuscitations	Thyroidectomy Vascular access	Parathyroidectomy Peripheral vascular Whipple
Post-op management	50% (all cases based if possible, allow the trainees to bring these cases to the group from their experience)	30%	30%	25%	20%

http://dx.doi.org/10.5772/intechopen.72120

ACGME competencies	PGY 1[1]	PGY 2	PGY 3	PGY 4	PGY 5
Fluid management	Routine fluid management				
Fever work-up	Work-up of fever at various times in the post-op period, use of imaging studies, use of lab tests, expected sources, appropriate treatment, appropriate communication	Direct the care of post-op patients	Anticipate post-operative needs	Direct post op management	Direct post-op management
Pain	End of Life curriculum				
Tubes, catheters	When to place and use, when to remove, how to monitor, how to place (skill), complications				
Mental status changes	Delirium, alcohol withdrawal, stroke, TIA, diabetic coma,				
Cardiopulmonary care	Hypertension, post-op pulmonary care, pneumonia, chest pain, management of tachycardia and bradycardia, CHF				
Wound management	Basic wound care, recognition of surgical site infections				
GI function	Ileus, constipation, stoma function and dysfunction, diarrhea, nausea and vomiting, PONV after anesthesia				
Complications	Oliguria, bowel obstruction, pulmonary embolus				
Practice-based learning and improvement					
EBM	Find articles relating to patient care problems	Question options in patient care	Define the options of care and begin to choose options	Know options of treatment and advantages and disadvantages	Establish own choices of patient management
Guidelines	Guideline and protocol development and use				

ACGME competencies	PGY 1[1]	PGY 2	PGY 3	PGY 4	PGY 5
Time management in OR	Understand time management in OR. Be on time for OR start times. Help get patient ready for the start time in OR.				
Outcomes/Outcomes Research/Quality	Understand structure, process, and outcome from a PI perspective	Be able to identify PI opportunities			
Personal Log Surgical learning and instructional portfolio (SLIP)	Complete and review 12/year in a portfolio format				
Adult learning	Apply learning principles to self	Apply to MS	Direct junior residents in their learning		
Teaching skills	Lecture preparation and presentation to peers, maybe even a videotape session, how to use PowerPoint presentation effectively, How to use visual aids when speaking to patients	MS clinical teaching		Resident clinical teach	Resident clinical teach
E-learning	As a learner: evaluate own strengths and weaknesses		Optimal use		
Interpersonal and communication skills					
Patient communication	Explain how operation will proceed the effect that pre-op management has on post-op complications		Telling bad news	Offer alternative treatments as part of consent	
	Be able to explain to a patient a procedure within their scope of practice, have a patient come in and have individuals practice on the individual.				
	Delivering bad news from EOL curriculum				
Professional communication	Develop approach to "hand-offs to colleagues				
Case presentation	Synthesize data and produce plan for scope of practice, Begin to keep case log on ACGME web site, introduction to coding of cases within scope of practice.				

ACGME competencies	PGY 1[1]	PGY 2	PGY 3	PGY 4	PGY 5
Informed Consent	What is Informed Consent, communicate to pt., document		Obtain consent routinely		
Medical writing	Dictations, discharge dictation content, letter writing, scientific writing		Direct junior residents in writing orders, write ICU orders	Manage an ICU plan	Direct overall patient care in any situation
Documentation	Importance of maintaining records in a timely fashion, coding and effect this has on billing for services.				
Medical error	How to share adverse events with patients and families, define medical error and its effects on healthcare				
Professionalism					
Principles (I-HEAARD)[3]	Integrity, honesty, excellence, altruism, accountability, respect, and duty				
Unprofessional behavior	Accountability: dealing with unprofessional behavior, know policy for disruptive physician				
	Duty to self - lifestyle - insurance - finance/ invest				
Medical License, Liability	Begin to work toward getting a Wisconsin medical license. Introduction to medical liability issues from MCWAH and malpractice carrier.			Coding exercise	JD exposure formal practice and practice management
Lifestyle	Understand the stresses of practice.	Helping colleagues		Leadership	Leadership
Mentoring	Role of a mentor			Become a mentor	
Systems-based practice[4]					
Societal issues and medicine	Case management. Be exposed to different healthcare systems. Discharge planning				

ACGME competencies	PGY 1[1]	PGY 2	PGY 3	PGY 4	PGY 5
Teamwork	Roles and responsibilities of personnel in ward care and in the OR, understand team management of patients	Understand the delegation of work	Begin to delegate		
Advocacy, medical liability	Organized medicine, belong to the candidate group of ACS, expert witness activity				Choose specialty group membership
Coordinate	Be a member of a team of caregivers		Organize a team of care givers		
Technology	Understand technology will drive medical costs, technology assessment tools, ProForma, ROI,			Identify when technology may be helpful	
Organizational structure	Quality management in health care systems, hospital administration and committee structure. Committee presentation and belong to committees		Understand PI principles		
Cost-effectiveness	Coding of personal cases, understand medical economics, understand economic terms		Cost breakdown by scope of practice	Cost breakdown by scope of practice	Cost breakdown by scope of practice
Safety	Understand drivers of error in medicine				

[1]Proficiency and Autonomy Expectation for exit PGY 1: The attending should be able to walk in the room and expect: a. Properly pre-op (e.g., position the patient). b. Reasonable level of understanding specific to scope of practice cases, which includes the steps (e.g., six ways to approach the umbilical/inguinal hernia repair – and associated EBM). c. Decide what step to do next. d. Perform with some guidance.

[2]When and how to use consultants preoperatively.

[3]ABIM –Acronym from Dept of Pediatrics at MCW: Integrity-Honesty, Excellence, Altruism, Accountability, Respect, Duty.

[4]SBP…requires that residents "demonstrate an awareness of and responsiveness to the larger context and system of health care and the ability to effectively call on system resources to provide care that is of optimal value" www.acgme.org/outcome/comp/comphome.asp. It includes understanding how their own practices affect others, and knowing how to partner with others to improve health care. Micro and macro (David Leach "No resident is an island" in Nov 2004 ACGME Bulletin pg. 2–3.

Table 3. Surgery curriculum blueprint developed by MCW Department of Surgery Curriculum Committee.

current PGY1 residents were better at handling their roles on clinical services. We were encouraged with our results and a decision was made to continue the PBC and expand it into the PGY2. Based on the feedback from the residents and services, the PGY1 curriculum was shortened to end on Thursday evening so that the PGY 1 residents could return to their services on Thursday rather than on Friday afternoon. Thus, the structure that continues to this day is Monday through Thursday as full days, with Sunday used to support preparation time.

2.2. Subsequent rollout and evaluation

On the basis of evaluations and feedback, the second year of implementation of the PGY1 PBC was formatted similar to the first year in regard to time commitment over the course of the year. Some topics were changed based on the evaluation feedback from residents and faculty. Since inception, each year the curriculum is reassessed and changed based on internal and external requests and feedback.

After the first year of the PBC roll out, the PGY2 curriculum was designed, and a Director was designated. This design used a similar model although shortened to full-day sessions Monday through Wednesday, with Sunday used for preparation and homework. The topics addressed came from our Curriculum blueprint. Changes included making appropriate accommodations for a different set of surgical procedures and increased responsibilities and expectations for our PGY2 residents. Each of the blocks in the PGY 2 year had a primary focus: trauma, critical care, vascular surgery, breast diseases, colorectal cancer, and diverticular disease. The sessions were focused on these broad areas within each block, though some topics covered spanned many diseases, such as professionalism, communication skills, among others. Again, feedback from residents and faculty has been positive despite the removal of residents from clinical service.

A curriculum was also designed for rollout the following year for the senior residents (PGY 3–5 curriculum) following the principles of protected time away from clinical duties and exams, but using a different structure and capturing many elements already in place such as skills labs for upper-level residents. Monthly half-day sessions were designed to cover multiple topics guided by surgical content in textbooks, skills sessions including open and laparoscopic surgery on pigs, simulator exercises, ethics sessions, and various topics to prepare residents for practice after graduation.

A Resident Curriculum Committee was formed and served to oversee the implementation and management of the curriculums, allowing a forum for discussing of outcomes, faculty recruitment for teaching opportunities, ideas for content, and challenges to overcome since the curriculums evolved. Eventually, the committee was no longer needed when the curriculums matured.

Our robust evaluation process for the PBC identified multiple expected and somewhat unanticipated benefits of this format. The residents improved in their medical knowledge. Comparison of preexams and postexams provided evidence of learning that was reproducible. A representative example is provided in **Figure 1**. American Board of Surgery In-Training Exam (ABSITE) scores of our PBC residents improved compared to our historical controls in our program. We found a statistically significant correlation of post-test curriculum exam scores early in the academic year

Team	Area/competency	Topics
Team C	Patient care	Order writing, pre-op assessments, use of consultants, perioperative management
Team D	Patient care/operative skills	Skills lab, instrument recognition, surgical technique
Team E	Medical knowledge/post-op management	Fluid management, fever work up, Pain management, tubes and catheters, mental status change, cardiopulmonary care, wound management, GI function, complications
Team F	Practice-based learning and improvement	EBM, guidelines, time management, Personal Logs (SLIPS), adult learning, teaching skills, E-learning
Team G	Interpersonal and communication skills	patient communication, professionalism communication, informed consent, medical writing, documentation, medical error
Team H	Professionalism	I-HEAARD, professional and unprofessional behavior, medical license
Team I	Systems-based practice	Societal issues and medicine, teamwork, advocacy, medical liability, safety

Table 4. Each area/competency was assigned specific topics. A faculty facilitator led a team of faculty to cover the material during sessions within the curriculum.

and yearly ABSITE scores, allowing the identification of resident exam performance concerns early in the year and providing time for improved ABSITE preparation [8]. The communication sessions with videotaping improved resident presentations at grand rounds and in our morbidity and mortality conferences [9]. Surgical skills based on PGY1 OSATS scores for suturing and knot tying were also significantly improved [10]. All these benefits were felt to be attributable to

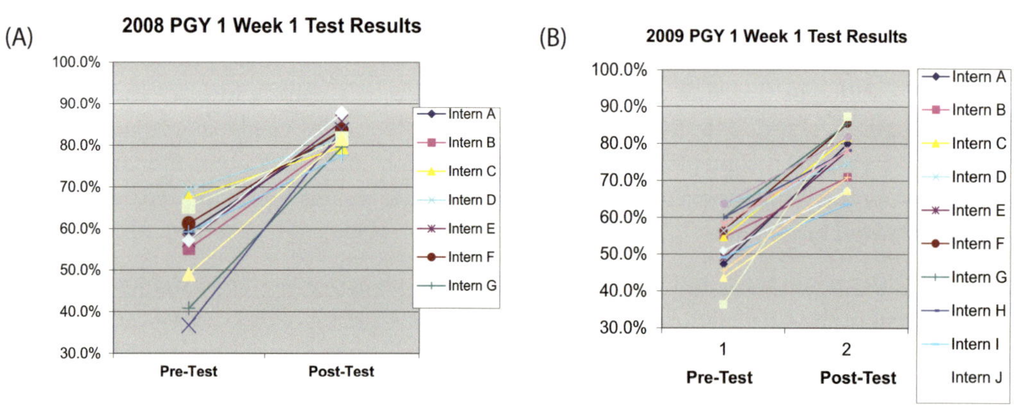

Figure 1. PGY 1 residents took the same written exam prior to the start of the curriculum session and again at the end of the session. Y-axis represents % correct. Depicted in (A) is a representative example of the highly variable knowledge set at the start of the curriculum week and the marked improvement at the end of the sessions. Depicted in (B) is the same results in the following year. Note that more residents from other surgical departments participated in the curriculum in the following year as depicted in B. The exams from year to year changed minimally and only to improve the clarity of questions based on analyses of the entire test and individual questions performed by MCW education services.

our curriculum presented in the PBC. Finally, importantly for physician wellness, the PBC format promoted a much closer collegiality among our PGY1 residents that, to this day, serves as a social support mechanism for each resident class throughout their training.

We also began to further analyze our results related to the infrastructure required to conduct the PBC [11]. Despite widespread support among department faculty, many faculty felt that the time and effort may not be worthwhile. This concern drove the Division of Education to complete a fiscal analysis of our PBC. We performed an assessment of the "costs" in hours and dollars for the protected block curriculum (PBC) for our PGY1 and PGY2 residents. Resources expended during the 2006–2007 academic year were evaluated in terms of the number, division, department, and rank of faculty involved in curriculum teaching. The hours of learner contact time and the monetary cost for consumable resources were calculated. The total number of faculty involved in the PGY1 curriculum was 49 compared to 29 for the PGY2 curriculum. Total faculty time spent teaching was 242.75 h (PGY1) and 156.5 h (PGY2) for 399.25 h. For both years of curriculum, total teaching hours by faculty rank within the Department of Surgery was 137.75 h for 12 assistant professors, 84.5 h for eight associate professors, 125.9 h for 15 professors, and 51.25 h for all others. Average time commitment for assistant professors was 11.5 h, for associate professors 10.7 h, and for professors 8.6 h ($p = 0.85$). Average time commitment for faculty in the Division of Education was 20.2 h, compared to 4.7 h for Departmental faculty in other divisions ($p = 0.0002$). The total monetary cost for consumable educational materials and space rental was $76,186. A dedicated educational curriculum in a surgical residency has substantial and real associated costs; however, we also felt that the benefits are well worth this effort.

A question of sustainable was also asked. We assessed results from our PGY1 and PGY2 PBC from 2005 to 2014. A total of 126 PGY 1 and 2 residents completed the PBC. The average number of contact hours for PGY1 residents was 175 and for PGY2 was 120. The total faculty time consumed was 508 h/year. The pre/post improvement averaged 15%. Our resident ratings continued to be greater than 4.5 over the 9 years, while the average faculty ratings were 4.6 on the five point scale. Our first time ABS pass rates for the qualifying exam (QE) improved after the entire resident cohort was enrolled in the PBC: 80% for pre-PBC-2005–2009 compared to 88% post-PBC-2010–2014. The most recent first time ABS QE pass rate from 2012 to 2016 has risen to 97%. These impressive pass rates support continued faculty and resident interest and commitment to sustain and evolve the curriculum.

2.3. Curriculum evolution

Over the past 12 years, our PBC for PGY1 and PGY2 residents has evolved. Since its initiation, resources on preparation for residency [12] recommended curriculum content [13], and basic and advanced surgery resident skills and procedures [14] have been made available. These resources, in addition to the new Surgical Council on Resident Education (SCORE) curriculum for General Surgery [15], serve to validate our own content and skills. Selected content from these resources has been incorporated into our curriculums, as appropriate. New graduation and American Board of Surgery requirements have led to the incorporation of the fundamentals of laparoscopic (FLS) and fundamentals of endoscopic (FES) curriculums as longitudinal elements of our curriculum content. Examples of the evolution of our PGY1 curriculum is shown in **Figure 2** with a representative sample of a typical day from 2006 compared to a typical week in 2016.

Our PBC remains highly rated by junior residents and faculty. It continues to evolve in content and duration as the department has expanded and health care delivery has changed. The

Time	Topic	Goals/Objectives
7:30-9:00	Diversity Training	1. Incorporate a patient centered approach in the daily care of patients 2. Identify ethnic and socio-economic barriers and disparities in health care
9:00-9:15	Break	
9:15-10:15	Video Case Review-Respiratory	1. Describe properties of gas exchange in health and disease 2. Identify spirometric lung volumes in health and disease 3. Choose appropriate vasopressors and inotropes in health and disease 4. Describe metabolic function(s) of the lung
10:15-10:30	Break	
10:30-11:30	Lecture-Basic Cardiac Physiology	1. The heart as a dual function chamber during systole and diastole 2. Laboratory and clinical evaluation of left ventricular systolic function 3. Application and limitations of clinical measures of left ventricular systolic function 4. Laboratory and clinical measurement of afterload 5. Definition and measurement of diastolic function 6. Role of diastolic function in cardiac pathophysiology and heart failure 7. Role of the left atrium in cardiac performance
11:30-12:45	Lunch	Sponsored by Pfizer Pharmaceuticals
12:45-2:00	Interactive CD-Stress Gastritis	1. Describe the pathophysiologic mechanisms involved in the development of stress-related mucosal bleeding and peptic ulcer disease bleeding 2. Explain the pharmacology, preparation, and administration of available therapeutic options preventing stress-related mucosal bleeding and peptic ulcer disease rebleeding in the critically ill patient 3. Outline the current applications of intravenous and oral acid-suppressive therapy in the critical care setting
2:00-3:45	Case Based Learning-Critical Care	1. Describe properties of gas exchange in health and disease 2. Identify spirometric lung volumes in health and disease 3. Choose appropriate vasopressors and inotropes in health and disease 4. Describe metabolic function(s) of the lung
3:45-4:00	Break	
4:00-5:00	Lecture-Ethics Committee	1. Describe two functions of an ethics committee 2. List four different potential members of an ethics committee
5:00	Debrief	

(A)

PGY 1 April 2016	Monday 18-Apr	Tuesday 19-Apr	Wednesday 20-Apr	Thursday 21-Apr	Friday 22-Apr
7:30 a.m. - 8:00 a.m.	PBL: Instruction & Self Taught Portion of Training Ventilator Associated Pneumonia *Carver*				
8:00 a.m. - 9:00 a.m.		Ethics Committee & Its Function *Morgenweck*	Nutrition & the Surgical Patient *Krzywda*	Evaluation & Surgical Management of Thyroid Disease *Carr*	
9:00 a.m. - 10:00 a.m.	**Case Presentations** Groups #3,4,5 *Redlich, Paul, Malinowski*	Patient Safety & Quality *Lamb*		Lower GI Bleed *Beckman*	
10:00 a.m. - 11:00 a.m.		Break Small Bowel Physiology & Inflammatory Bowel Disease *Otterson*	Patient Centered Care/Cultural Competency *Webb*	Basic Science *Kugler*	
11:00 a.m. - 12:00 p.m.		Burns *Sato*	Bugs & Drugs *Graham*	PBL Review Session: VAP *Carver*	
12:00 p.m. - 1:00 p.m.	Ventilators 101 *Paul*			**Loupe Fitting** *Designs for Vision*	
1:00 p.m. - 2:00 p.m.	ENDO TOWER **Groups A & B** *Procedure Rm 4* Ultrasound *STAR Center Rm:2710* **Group C** *Carver* CVL *STAR Center Rm:2710* **Group D** *Malinowski; Paul*	ENDO TOWER **GROUPS C & D** *Procedure Rm 4* Ultrasound *STAR Center Rm:2710* **Group A** *Carver* CVL *STAR Center Rm:2710* **Group B** *Malinowski; Paul*	IHI Modules *Mila*		
2:00 p.m. - 3:00 p.m.	FEC **Group A** *Kastenmeier* FLS **Group B** *Higgins*	FEC **Group C** *Kastenmeier* FLS **Group D** *Higgins*	**Pig Colon Stapling Lab** *Ridolfi, Peterson*	Mock Oral Scenarios *Malinowski*	
3:00 p.m. - 4:00 p.m.	CVL *STAR Center Rm:2710* **Group C** *Malinowski; Paul* Ultrasound *STAR Center Rm:2710* **Group D** *Carver* FLS **Group A** *Higgins* FEC **Group B** *Kastenmeier*	CVL *STAR Center Rm:2710* **Group A** *Malinowski; Paul* Ultrasound *STAR Center Rm:2710* **Group B** *Carver* FLS **Group C** *Higgins* FEC **Group D** *Kastenmeier*		Session Evaluation/ Feedback Session	
4:00 p.m. - 5:00 p.m.				*Return to Service*	

(B)

Figure 2. Depicted is a selected schedule of the PGY 1 curriculum from 2006 (A) (one of 4 days) and 2017 (B) (all 4 days). Note the types of didactic sessions in (A) compared to a mix of didactic and skills-based sessions (in dark gray) including those that address the new FLS and FEC requirements in (B).

program is now 4.5 days (Monday through Thursday, Sunday afternoon for final preparation) for PGY1 and 3.5 days (Monday through Wednesday, Sunday afternoon for final preparation) for PGY2 residents. Whether the reduction in time is related to an improvement in preparation of medical students for residency or our concern over clinical exposure is an unanswered question. We do believe that the presence of the PBC has had a positive impact on resident recruitment as it demonstrates our emphasis and dedication to surgical education. Anecdotally, some residents have expressed their interest in our PBC and opportunities for educational research as reasons for choosing our residency training programs.

The success of the program for the PGY1 residents has some local external validity of importance. We were asked by the Departments of Plastic and Urologic Surgery to include their residents in the program. These program directors recognized the potential positive impact on their junior residents as well. This inclusion helps bonding among residents who will be closely working together throughout their training program.

We have also continued to improve the separate educational sessions for our PGY3–5 curriculum. This curriculum was started in 2007 and replaced a straight didactic lecture series. It is held on one Wednesday morning, which is currently transitioning to Friday mornings, each month for 4 h providing 32 h of contact time. Again, the residents are relieved from clinical duty. A faculty facilitator leads discussion topics. These sessions are case based and the format is very similar to oral board questioning. These changes were requested by our residents as they became familiar with the PGY1 and PGY2 curriculums. The topics cycle every 3 years. Sessions on ethics are included.

Another addition added to our PGY1 and 2 PBC was surgical jeopardy. This has become a favorite for a few faculty facilitators as well as for our residents. This type of interactive game-based instruction has been utilized to teach and provide a casual, fun environment for residents to compete and socialize [16]. We participate in the American College of Surgeons (ACS) resident jeopardy session at the annual ACS Clinical Congress meeting. While we have never taken the top prize at the ACS Clinical Congress Jeopardy competition, we have been competitive many times.

Finally, the PBC has been a venue for scholarship for faculty interested in surgical education. A number of PBC-related manuscripts and presentations regarding our PBC curriculum have been published in peer-reviewed journals and in the AAMC MedEdPORTAL, respectively. Having a robust, sustainable, evolving, and faculty-supported curriculum has allowed many faculty, and selected residents, to pursue surgical education as a component of their careers interests. The current PGY1 curriculum director is enrolled in a Masters of Education in the Health Professions program and the PGY 2 curriculum director is enrolled in the Association for Surgical Education (ASE) Surgical Education Research Fellowship.

3. Conclusions

Surgical education requires constant attention and new methods of teaching and assessment must be considered. The PBC was initially met with a significant amount of skepticism from some faculty and senior residents resistant to change. However, as residents experienced the new model, it was uniformly accepted and ultimately highly valued by the department. We believe that maintaining a positive focus on the educational mission allowed us to accomplish such a change to the traditional delivery of resident education. As the skills needed by health care providers continue to change, so must our educational objectives and how we deliver them. Our PBC has allowed us to focus on these new skills and competencies and provided a venue for continued evolution as we look to the future. Faculty interested in careers in surgical education makes the curriculum sustainable and ensures future scholarly products studying educational outcomes of our curriculums and surgical training programs.

3.1. Future of the PBC

We will continue to look for ways to improve our PBC. We are convinced that the learning environment we have established for our trainees is more conducive to the educational needs of our residents. Being away from clinical service allows their focus to be on learning and more receptive to learning without the distractions of clinical care. How we balance educational time and clinical service will need continuous evaluation and adjustment to meet the needs of our trainees.

Potential areas of future change that need ongoing evaluation relate to educational objectives and the needs of our trainees. Educational objectives will need to address the multitude of changes in medicine that continue to occur. These include the application of advanced medical devices, use of alternative interventions to surgery, medical care organizational changes, and quality and safety initiatives. While newer topics must be addressed, we also must not let them displace critical basic medical knowledge, patient care principles and basic skills common to surgical practice.

As our trainees transition from millennials to generation Zs, our educational techniques will need to change. A generation of learners raised with Internet access, social media, and mobile access will force us to consider how we deliver our material. Classroom time may decrease as mobile active learning opportunities increase. Manipulating the PBC into this type of learning should not be difficult, but it will require thoughtful planning.

Regardless of the changes required, we believe the infrastructure that we have designed will be flexible and sturdy enough to meet these challenges.

Author details

Philip N. Redlich[1,2], Travis P. Webb[1,3] and John A. Weigelt[1*]

*Address all correspondence to: jweigelt@mcw.edu

1 Department of Surgery, Medical College of Wisconsin, Milwaukee, Wisconsin, United States

2 Surgical Care Division, Clement J. Zablocki VA Medical Center, Milwaukee, Wisconsin, United States

3 Academic Affairs, Medical College of Wisconsin, Milwaukee, Wisconsin, United States

References

[1] Kotter JP. Learning Change. Boston, MA: Harvard Business School Press; 1996

[2] http://www.absurgery.org/xfer/curriculumoutline2017-18_book.pdf. Accessed September 2017

[3] https://www.facs.org/education/program/resident-skills. Accessed September 2017

[4] http://www.acgme.org/Portals/0/PDFs/Milestones/SurgeryMilestones.pdf. Accessed September 2017

[5] http://www.acgme.org/Specialties/Documents-and-Resources/pfcatid/24/Surgery. Accessed September 2017

[6] Webb TP, Weigelt JA, Redlich PN, Andersen RC, Brasel KJ, Simpson D. Protected block curriculum enhances learning during general surgery residency training. Archives of Surgery. Feb 2009;**144**(2):160-166

[7] Webb TP, Aprahamian C, Weigelt JA, Brasel KJ. The surgical learning and instructional portfolio (SLIP) as a self-assessment educational tool demonstrating practice-based learning. Current Surgery. November–December 2006;**63**(6):444-447

[8] Webb TP, Paul J, Treat R, Codner P, Anderson R, Redlich P. Surgery residency curriculum examination scores predict future American Board of Surgery in-Training Examination Performance. Journal of Surgical Education. September/October 2014;**71**(5):743-747

[9] Gribovskaja-Rupp I, Redlich P, Treat R, Webb T, Anderson R. Teaching oral and PowerPoint skills for the surgical morbidity and mortality (M&M) conference presentation. MedEdPORTAL. 2013 Available from: www.mededportal.org/publication/9338

[10] Wade TJ et al. The Journal of Surgical Research. 2012 Jun 05;**181**(1):1-5

[11] Webb TP, Brasel KJ, Redlich PN, Weigelt JA. Putting a price on education: Hours and dollars for a general surgery curriculum. American Journal of Surgery. 2010;**199**:126-130

[12] https://www.facs.org/education/program/fsc

[13] https://www.facs.org/education/division-of-education/publications/navigatefirstyear

[14] https://www.facs.org/education/program/resident-skills

[15] http://portal.surgicalcore.org

[16] Webb TP, Simpson D, Denson S, Duthie E. Gaming used as an informal instructional technique: Effects on learner knowledge and satisfaction. Journal of Surgical Education. May 2012;**69**(3):330-334

Chapter 5

Virtual and Augmented Reality in Medical Education

Panteleimon Pantelidis, Angeliki Chorti,
Ioanna Papagiouvanni, Georgios Paparoidamis,
Christos Drosos, Thrasyvoulos Panagiotakopoulos,
Georgios Lales and Michail Sideris

Additional information is available at the end of the chapter

http://dx.doi.org/10.5772/intechopen.71963

Abstract

Virtual reality (VR) and augmented reality (AR) are two contemporary simulation models that are currently upgrading medical education. VR provides a 3D and dynamic view of structures and the ability of the user to interact with them. The recent technological advances in haptics, display systems, and motion detection allow the user to have a realistic and interactive experience, enabling VR to be ideal for training in hands-on procedures. Consequently, surgical and other interventional procedures are the main fields of application of VR. AR provides the ability of projecting virtual information and structures over physical objects, thus enhancing or altering the real environment. The integration of AR applications in the understanding of anatomical structures and physiological mechanisms seems to be beneficial. Studies have tried to demonstrate the validity and educational effect of many VR and AR applications, in many different areas, employed via various hardware platforms. Some of them even propose a curriculum that integrates these methods. This chapter provides a brief history of VR and AR in medicine, as well as the principles and standards of their function. Finally, the studies that show the effect of the implementation of these methods in different fields of medical training are summarized and presented.

Keywords: virtual reality, augmented reality, medical education, simulation, advanced learning

1. Introduction

Virtual reality (VR) and augmented reality (AR) are the current trends in medical education. VR is the virtual construction of an artificial world. The key element of VR is the high level of user's immersion over the virtual environment, namely, the high level of structures' fidelity, as well as the interaction of the user with them in a realistic manner. This has become recently available, as it requires high standards of certain technologies, including advanced haptic devices with force-feedback capabilities (bidirectional stimuli), high-resolution audio-visual effects, motion detection technology, and high-performance processing power to transmit, and processes all this information with near-zero latency.

The first virtual system in medicine was introduced in 1965 by Robert Mann, in order to facilitate a new training environment for orthopedic. In the late 1980s, the head-mounted display (HMD) was introduced as a wearable device for VR visualizations in medicine [1]. The first pioneering applications in medical education were some on hands-on procedures that appeared over a decade later [2, 3]. In the 1990s, many adverse effects from the use of VR were reported. Nausea, dizziness, temporarily impaired vision, and lack in the sense of presence, even after 20 min of use, were some of them. The adverse effects were attributed to technical defects, such as the lag time and the inability of the human eye to fixate in-depth to "artificially distant" 3D objects [4, 5]. Although these effects are minor and subside quickly nowadays, the risk of learning inappropriate handling moves, when low-fidelity or badly simulated models are used and particularly under unsupervised teaching, still remains [6].

Although AR and VR share many technical aspects, AR differs from VR as its target is not to construct a fully artificial environment but to overlay computer-generated images onto images of the real world [7]. Therefore, it uses machines that allow physical view of the surrounding environment to be visible but enhanced with virtual images. Tablets, mobile phones, AR glasses, and other optimized devices can be employed as hardware for running AR applications. Historically, the development of AR starts in the 1960s, but the term "augmented reality" was established in 1990. The increase in the use of AR came along with the technological advances that made it available and useful. Nowadays, AR is used widely in the clinical setting, providing extra information for the clinician during interventional procedures (CT/MRI guidance, visualization of paths), but it is also applied in the educational world. Anatomy, with the 3D visualization of hardly comprehensible structures, and physiology, with the representation of mechanisms in 4D (in space and time dimensions), are the main areas of interest [8].

2. Technical aspects

VR and AR come with certain hardware requirements in order to retain high standards of simulation. The computerized 3D pictures and audio have to be realistic and simulate both real and abstract structures. The motion of the user should be detected with high precision so that the visual field (size, shape, angle of objects) and auditory stimuli (volume, sound balance) can change accordingly. The user must be able to affect the virtual environment but also to be affected via haptic feedback stimuli. Haptic devices, such as joysticks, gloves, and other specialized tools, serve these haptic interaction needs. High-performance computer power is needed to process the huge amount of information produced, with low, unnoticeable latency. All these contribute to the key element of VR and AR: immersion of the user over the environment. Moreover, fast and reliable Internet connection is needed to support the latest trend in VR field, namely, the establishment of VR fora where users meet and interact with each other online, in a common virtual environment [1, 3, 9].

Many VR settings involve HMD. HMD is a wearable device that offers visualization of the constructed virtual reality in wide angle and does not permit the disturbance of the virtual experience by external visual stimuli. Although the first HMDs had a restricted resolution of 800 × 600 pixels and a narrow vision angle of 30°, the current HMDs display fully high-definition images, with angles that can reach 360°. Some of them are wireless and may incorporate position and motion detection systems for the eye and head movements. Although HMDs play a significant role in many VR settings, they are not mandatory for all medical applications. The simulation of many procedures, such as laparoscopic or endoscopic, requires the display of the virtual images on a computer screen [10]. Sound quality is also important for a complete VR experience. Volume and balance adjustments according to the moves of the users are significant elements of the VR environment [1].

Input devices consist of all the devices that transmit the user's stimuli to the VR system. Gloves, joysticks, or other specialized tools (laparoscopic or endoscopic instruments) are usually employed. A special subcategory of necessary input devices for VR is sensors and trackers. Sensors and trackers identify the position and the direction of the user in space as an input stimulus, allowing interaction. They employ various technologies such as lasers, infrared radiation, and mechanical detectors and can detect the properties of the whole body, the head, or even the subtle gestures and moves of the hands, ability that is extremely useful in medical procedures' simulation. The recent technological improvement of these devices, which made the VR setting suitable for medical training, is the tactile-feedback ability. Adjusted force is exerted via the handling instruments, depending on the hand moves. Thus, the operator has a more realistic, bidirectional haptic experience when performing a virtual surgical process or other interventional processes [10].

Most AR hardware use glasses that project virtual 3D images onto the real environment. While *Google Glass* and *Epson Smart Glasses* were the pioneering devices, newer devices, such as *Hololens* (*Microsoft*), combine AR glasses with a system of tracking cameras and sensors. Tablets are an alternative platform suitable for AR applications. While the camera captures the physical world, virtual structures are added in the screen [10].

3. Quality control and educational impact

VR and AR simulators must possess quality standards so as to be suitable for medical education purposes. However, even if these standards are met, the educational benefit is still not guaranteed a priori. There are many published studies that try to test VR and AR simulators in specific educational settings (concerning different medical fields and stages of training) in order to examine their validity, the transferability of the taught skills to the real world, the acceleration of the learning curve, and the retention period of the skills. Following the determination of these parameters, establishing a curriculum that integrates this evidence in a productive and cost-efficient manner is an essential consequence.

High-resolution images, quality in sound, haptic input and feedback devices, and high processing power are the parameters that are required to create realistic VR/AR environment. Moreover, the structures of the organs and tissues must be of high fidelity, and the change in their shape, size, and angle of view must correspond completely to the user's moves and handlings. Otherwise, there is a risk that the moves and skills learnt will be inappropriate in real situations [6]. ISO criteria have also been established. They include initial assessment of the educational needs and establishment of a technical solution. This requires the in-depth knowledge of the procedures or mechanisms that will be simulated. After the concept generation, the setting must be validated, in order to examine if it meets the educational expectations. Moreover, technical experts, medical experts, representatives from end-user groups, human factor experts, and designers should collaborate and form an interdisciplinary team that will design, evaluate, and upgrade the VR/AR products [11, 12].

Furthermore, VR and AR systems meeting these standards have to undergo post-market validation studies, in order to examine if they provide the educational effect they are expected to. In terms of medical education, the studies examine the following types of validity: (1) face validity—usually the end users make subjective comments as feedback for the quality and realism of the setting. (2) Content validity: once again, it is subjectively defined by the users' comments but with emphasis to the content of the simulation (procedures, fidelity of organs, etc.). (3) Construct validity: this employs objective statistical methods that aim to correlate the actual skill level of the participants with their performance in the VR setting. Usually, there are two or more groups that differ only to the level of skills. Their performance in the VR/AR setting is evaluated, either by external human evaluators or, if it is feasible, by the VR system itself. If there is a correlation, that means that the VR setting can effectively discriminate between novices and experienced users. This is extremely useful when using VR/AR settings as assessment tools for the progress of trainees, as they provide an objective evaluation that may not require the need of human evaluators. (4) Concurrent validity: another objective validity control that aims to correlate the performance in the VR/AR setting with other existing evaluation tools. This practically checks whether the VR/AR evaluation results point to the same direction with other evaluation tools that are considered as gold standards. (5) Predictive validity: the last but probably most useful objective validity control. Two homogenous cohorts of trainees are formed. After that, only one receives a specific VR/AR training, with predefined parameters (such as the simulator model, the procedure/topic learnt, the time, the frequency and the difficulty level of the procedure, and the presence of a supervisor). On the contrary, the other cohort receives training with differently optimized parameters (perhaps another VR/AR simulator or even a completely different simulation method) or does not receive training at all and is used as a control group. Subsequently, the skills of both cohorts are evaluated in real patients or other simulation settings that are considered as gold standards with proven discriminating ability. If a correlation exists, the VR setting can have an educational effect that can be indeed transferred to real patients. Some studies evaluate the effect of the training after a long time period to examine the retention period of the skills [8, 13].

If there is confirmed predictive validity of a VR/AR simulator for acquiring a specific skill set, then the next step is to wonder: "How much does the VR/AR training contribute to the acceleration of the acquired skills?" This is a more complex question that can be approached with learning curves. A learning curve is a graph that correlates the level of acquired skills with the amount of effort exerted (measured in time, number of trials or procedures performed). In general, it is desired that the learning curve has a high plateau, meaning that the final level of skills acquired with this method will be high, but also is steep, meaning that there is an early high acceleration of skills with little effort. If a trainee that has completed the training in the VR setting (namely, he/she has reached the plateau of the VR/AR learning curve) and then is able to receive training in other settings (e.g., other simulation settings or real patients) from a higher than the basic level, then we assume that the VR/AR training offers transferable skills and has "accelerated" the learning curve. The common characteristics of the learning curves on most VR/AR simulators are the low plateau, the transferability of the skills, and the steep shape. Low plateau means that the total level of skills that can be acquired is lower than the one with other education methods; thus, the VR/AR is usually appropriate for novices, but is not of any significant benefit for more experienced users. Fortunately, it usually has a steep shape and transferability properties, meaning that these skills are acquired quickly and then can be transferred to other education settings. In other words, VR/AR training compensates for some training period in the initial steps of other educational settings.

After these VR/AR setting-specific properties are evaluated, the next step is to define a curriculum that incorporates VR/AR methods in education. This curriculum must also take into account the cost of both VR/AR and alternative ways of training, as well as the patient risk for both settings. For example, if there is a high risk in training with real patients or high cost with animal-simulation models, a VR/AR simulator (with low plateau and steep learning curve) can compensate quickly for the initial steps, offering a safe, relatively inexpensive, and reproducible alternative choice that may provide transferrable skills.

As there are many validation and evaluating studies in literature, an overall profile of VR/AR applications can be formed. In general, it seems that VR offers an appropriate environment for training in hands-on procedures. As **Table 1** shows, laparoscopic surgery, neurosurgery, catheterization techniques, and endoscopic procedures seem to be the main fields of VR applications. Novices are the most benefited trainees, while there is not a significant learning effect in experienced users. VR offers great diversity with only one setting. The educational setting can be reproducible with a variety of different optimization details, not restricted by the physical world [1]. Although VR simulators are expensive to purchase, they can be used recurrently with low cost, require less staff than other methods (animal models or real patients), and guarantee no risk for the patient [8, 12]. However, there are certain disadvantages in their use. In the common case of crashing, the virtual experience is destroyed. From a technical point of view, they are still not ready to present a virtual environment with absolute fidelity, as if

Fields of educational training	VR and AR simulator examples
Physiology and anatomy	Visible Human Project, Visible Korean Human, The Virtual Body, The Virtual Human Embryo, The Visible Human Server, AR glasses, mobile phone and tablet based AR applications
Open surgery	Virtual Reality Educational Surgical Tools
Laparoscopic surgery	MIST-VR, LaparoscopyVR™, LapMentor™, LapSim™, SINERGIA, Xitact LS500®, ProMIS®
Robotic surgery	RoSS™, DV-Trainer®, SEP Robot, da Vinci Skills Simulator (dVSS) ™
Oesophagogastroduodenoscopy, colonoscopy, ERCP	GI Mentor™, EndoVR™, Olympus Endo TS-1
Neurosurgery	NeuroVR (NeuroTouch, NeuroTouch Cranio)™, ImmersiveTouch®, RoboSim, Vascular Intervention Simulation Trainer®, EasyGuide Neuro, ANGIO Mentor™, VIVENDI, Dextroscope®, Anatomical Simulator for Pediatric Neurosurgery
Interventional cardiology and cardiothoracic surgery	ANGIO Mentor™, Vascular Intervention Simulation Trainer (VIST)®, Vimedix (equipped with Hololens) ™, Nakao Cardiac Model, Minimally Invasive Cardiac Surgery Simulator, dVSS™, EchoCom
Urology	URO Mentor™, University of Washington TURP Trainer, UROSim™, PelvicVisionTURP simulator, GreenLight laser simulator, Kansai HoLEP, ProMIS®
Orthopedics	ImmersiveTouch®, Phantom haptics interface®, Gaumard HAL S2001® and S3000® Mannequins, Novint Falcon®, Medtronic model, Arthro-VR®, Arthro MENTOR™, ArthroSIM, ArthroS™
Endovascular surgery	ANGIO Mentor™, Vascular Intervention Simulation Trainer (VIST)®, Cardio CT, SimSuite, Compass 2™
Obstetrics and gynecology	HystSim™, EssureSim™, AccuTouch (and newly version from CAE Healthcare), MIST-VR, LapSim™
ENT	OtoSim™, VOXEL-MAN (supports Phantom haptics), Ohio State University surgical simulator, Stanford Surgical Simulator, Mediseus, ImmersiveTouch, Endoscopic Sinus Surgery Simulator (supports Phantom haptics), Dextroscope®, dVSS ™
Ophthalmology	EyeSi®, MicrovisTouch™, PhacoVision®
Intubation and bronchoscopy	EndoVR Simulator™, BRONCH Mentor™, ORSIM®

Table 1. VR and AR simulator examples with respect to each educational field.

it was real. Last but not least, wrong handling can be learnt, particularly under unsupervised learning. The VR simulators can reconstruct a whole virtual surgery, specific procedural tasks, or even more abstract procedures [2].

Moreover, many of the simulators have incorporated assessment tools of the user's performance. They evaluate parameters like path distance, operation time, moves, and errors and then deliver quantified, timely, and objective metrics. If these simulators meet construct validity criteria, they can be used to objectively assess the trainee's performance. However, if this ability is not supported, human experts can also play the role of the evaluator, and studies have also shown acceptable metrics [8].

Although AR finds many clinical applications in medicine, its implementation in medical education is not so extensive (see **Table 1**). However, tablets and mobile phones have AR applications that enrich traditional reading with pop-up videos, links, and interactive material [14]. Moreover, in medical training there are AR applications that project traumas and other lesions onto healthy humans, aiming at training students and residents in the management of these situations. However, interventional procedures are not performed, and the AR applications are restricted in teaching the theoretical context of these subjects in an increased reality setting [15].

4. Applications in educational fields

4.1. Preclinical teaching

Anatomy and physiology are the classic paradigms that have the majority of VR/AR applications [6]. A checkpoint in the development of VR/AR applications that study human structures and mechanisms is the construction of massive online databases that contain human images and information, mostly obtained with CT/MRI scanning. The first relevant project, called the *Visible Human Project*, was created by the University of Colorado in 1991. The male and female versions of the project contain over 7000 digital anatomical images and occupy over 50 gigabytes of space. The National Library of Medicine made this platform free and accessible [6, 16]. Other similar models followed, such as the Korean model *Visible Korean Human*, *The Virtual Body*, *The Virtual Human Embryo*, and *The Visible Human Server*. Anatomy teaching was enhanced with VR applications that obtained data from these databases. Similar effort was put to reconstruct intracellular organelles in physiology [2, 10]. Structures and mechanisms are digitally simulated and presented in four dimensions (space and time). This contemporary visualization can be called "in silico" biology. Examples include the dynamic simulation of neurons, membranes, and cardiovascular system parameters including heart rate, blood pressure, contractility, and vascular resistance [16]. Anatomy also uses tablet-/smartphone-based AR applications that project extensive information, visual 3D structures, and links onto the traditional pages of anatomy textbooks. Recently, other hardware platforms, such as the *Hololens* glasses by Microsoft, started to support relevant applications [19]. An application allows the interactive, 3D exploration of the human brain, reconstructed with MRI data. Hand gestures allow the deformation, fly-by view, and other interactions with the 3D model to reveal hidden organs [10].

4.2. Surgery

VR and AR find most of their applications in surgery and particularly in laparoscopic surgery training. Endoscopic procedures and neurosurgery are also popular. Fidelity and realism are extremely important factors in these fields, not only for the comfort of the user but also for guaranteeing that no improper handling will be learnt and that the actual stressful conditions will be recreated. VR/AR simulators demonstrate certain advantages, such the minimal cost per use, the absence of ethical issues, and the safety compared to training on actual patients. Moreover, greater diversity and complexity in the procedures can be achieved. However, the cost of purchasing and maintaining is high, and also despite the rapid advances in VR/AR technologies, the realism still fails in representing the operating room settings with high fidelity [17].

4.2.1. Laparoscopic surgery

The current VR laparoscopic simulators are characterized as "hybrid" as they have real instruments and a virtual operating field, projected on a screen or other display devices. They provide haptic feedback to users according to their handlings, and most of them have assessment systems that measure parameters such as the time to complete a task, the errors made during surgery, and the surgeon's economy of movements. They can have both "task trainer" modules, for training in more simple and abstract handlings, and also "complete operation" modules that simulate the whole operating procedure [18]. They seem to benefit the novices, especially when intensive feedback by the instructor is applied [19]. The following simulators are among the most popular:

Minimally Invasive Surgical Trainer-Virtual Reality (*MIST-VR, Wolfson Centre and VR Solutions*): it provides a 3D environment for practicing abstract tasks and moves with a cylinder and a ball. It can be adjusted to six difficulty levels, and it can teach basic laparoscopic skills like suturing and knot tying. It is a low-fidelity simulator that does not support force-feedback function [18, 20]. It has demonstrated construct validity but controversial transferability of skills [21, 22].

LaparoscopyVR™ (*LapVR™, Immersion*): this simulator supports haptic hardware for force-feedback function. Studies show that inexperienced surgeons acquire skills that can be transferred in real procedures. *LapVR™* system allows both individual and team training and offers training in six basic handlings with adjustable levels of difficulty: camera navigation, using the hook electrode, cutting, clipping, suturing, and knot tying. It also has a module for laparoscopic cholecystectomy with 18 alternative cases and 3 levels of difficulty. It also contains a module for ectopic pregnancy, tubal occlusion, and adnexa's pathology [2, 20].

LapMentor™ (*3D Systems, formerly Simbionix*): it targets both novices and experienced surgeons, teaching from basic laparoscopic skills to complete laparoscopic operations. It also has an incorporated assessment system for providing metrics to the user. It is characterized by high fidelity and the ability to provide haptic feedback. The modules include basic laparoscopic skills, suturing, laparoscopic cholecystectomy, ventral hernia, gastric bypass, and gynecology cases. Information on handling tissue, handling tools, time, and movement efficiency are obtained during the simulation and are processed to produce metrics [2, 20]. It has demonstrated construct validity, predictive validity, and transferability of technical skills, especially when combined with supervision by the instructors [21, 23].

LapSim™ (*Surgical Science*): this system includes basic skill modules, anastomosis and suture scenarios, and laparoscopic cholecystectomy scenarios, and one case is dedicated to gynecology.

It is a high-fidelity simulator with the ability of transferring functions between instructors and institutions. It has shown good construct and predictive validity and transferability of some skills [2, 18, 20, 21].

The sustainability of the skills obtained with VR simulators is supported by few studies with small samples and a short follow-up period [24]. Other VR/AR models are *SINERGIA*, *Xitact LS500®* (*Xitact*), and *ProMIS®* (*Haptica*) [13, 20, 21].

The main application of AR in laparoscopic surgical training is telementoring: the supervisor can teach the trainee by indicating the proper surgical moves, paths, and handlings on the AR screen. These pieces of information are displayed to the trainee and guide them [25]. However, research has shown that this might also distract the user. A study proposes displaying this information on an additional sub-monitor, rather than on a single head-up display [26].

4.2.2. Robotic surgery

RoSS™ (*Simulated Surgical Systems*) and *DV-Trainer®* (*Mimic Technologies*) are robotic surgery VR trainers that have shown face and content validity. *DV-Trainer®*, along with *SEP Robot* (*SimSurgery*) and *da Vinci Skills Simulator™* (*dVSS™*, *Intuitive Surgical*), provides metrics about the trainees' performance with construct validity. *RoSS™* is the only one that incorporates whole procedural tasks [27].

As the current robotic surgery systems do not rely on tactile feedback, their simulators are also freed from this need. However, for educational purposes an alteration in color in the surgical field exists, depending on the force that the users apply. Training in robotic surgery with VR simulators seems to provide better and transferable surgical skills, as shown by some studies [28, 29]. Novices are found to be particularly benefited from training in robotic simulators [30].

4.2.3. Open surgery

There is a limited variety in open surgery VR simulators and a lack of validation studies, probably because the complexity and the hands-on nature (without the involvement of machine systems) of open surgery operations do not provide an easily simulated environment. *Virtual Reality Educational Surgical Tools* (*VREST*) has developed an open surgery simulator for training and assessment. It consists of two haptic devices with haptic feedback enabled and a system that represents 3D images. The software allows the optimization of the scenarios from the teacher. The trainees decide what instruments to use and are assessed by the machine. The first module built on the *VREST* platform was an inguinal hernia repair according to Lichtenstein. Another similar simulator was developed by the Imperial College London, which has shown construct validity [31].

4.3. Endoscopic procedures

4.3.1. Oesophagogastroduodenoscopy (OGD)

GI Mentor™ (*3D Systems, formerly Simbionix*) is the only validated VR simulator for upper endoscopy training. Although beneficial for novices, it is of limited benefit for the experienced users. Procedure time, time to reach specific landmarks, intubation time, movement techniques, procedural success rates, and other patient-related outcomes are evaluated in metrics. Studies show that trainees have a significantly lower overall procedure time and a significantly improved technical accuracy, compared to controls [32].

4.3.2. Colonoscopy

More VR simulators are available for colonoscopy training. The evidence that supports the use of VR trainers in the early stages of training is well established. The repetitions required to reach the plateau of VR training are 7–10, depending on the study. After this checkpoint there must be a switch to traditional endoscopy training. The combination of these two methods has been found more beneficial than either of the two alone. The skills acquired with VR training were maintained for at least 9 months [33]. *GI Mentor™*, *EndoVR™* (*CAE Healthcare, the old AccuTouch®, Immersion*) and *Olympus Endo TS-1* (*Olympus*) are among the simulators that have been studied and have showed construct and predictive validity [21, 33]. *GI Mentor™* has been chosen by SAGES as the platform for the Fundamentals of Endoscopic Surgery™ (FES™) examination [34].

4.3.3. Endoscopic retrograde cholangiopancreatography (ERCP)

GI Mentor™ (*3D Systems, formerly Simbionix*) is the only validated simulator for ERCP among six devices in total. It has been found to be beneficial in acquiring transferable skills and to have the potential to be included in training programs, although it lacks in terms of realism, usefulness, and performance compared to bench model trainers [32, 35]. *EndoVR™* is another popular simulator with ERCP modules available.

4.4. Neurosurgery

Neurosurgery training is a field where VR and AR simulators are usually found. Such simulators must be comfortable enough to wear for many hours; extremely realistic, so that they represent effectively the detailed neurosurgery structures; and affordable [36]. They demonstrate several advantages when compared to physical models (animal or bench models): they have a lower cost in use, there is no limit in the repetitions, and they offer a great sense of variety and diversity in the simulated cases. However, the resolution and realism of the constructed world are still issues to be resolved [37].

NeuroVR™ (*CAE Healthcare*): a neurosurgical training platform that simulates microdissections, tumor aspiration, and hemostasis. It was first introduced as *NeuroTouch*, a platform designed from over 50 experts from the National Research Council Canada [18]. It provides complex computer-generated metrics in 13 categories; thus it is suitable for use as assessment tool. As there seems to be a plateau in acquired skills, the educational benefit may be limited to early learners. Other specialized variations of the simulator also exist, such as the *NeuroTouch Cranio*, a simulator for brain tumor resection. The trainer provides haptic feedback and measures the trainee's performance [37].

ImmersiveTouch® (*ImmersiveTouch*) is an AR simulator used for training in many surgical disciplines, including spine surgery, neurosurgery, ENT surgery, and ophthalmology [13].

It consists of two physical instruments, which can simulate various surgical instruments, and a system that projects the virtual surgical field onto the hands and the instruments of the user in an interactive way. It was found a valid training method for thoracic pedicle screw placement (face and predictive validity) and clipping aneurysms (face validity) but also for percutaneous trigeminal rhizotomy (construct validity) [13, 38]. Moreover, it had positive learning effect and can accelerate the learning curve in many neurosurgical procedures, such as ventriculostomy, vertebroplasty, and finding the anatomical landmarks for various interventional techniques [39, 40].

Various other VR/AR simulators exist. *RoboSim, Vascular Intervention Simulation Trainer®* (*VIST®, Mentice*), *EasyGuide Neuro* (*Philips Medical Systems*), *ANGIO Mentor™* (*3D Systems, formerly Simbionix*), *VIVENDI* (*University of Tübingen, Germany*), *Dextroscope®* (*Bracco AMT*), and *Anatomical Simulator for Pediatric Neurosurgery* (*ASPN, Pro Delphus*) are commercially or academically developed systems that simulate solely neurosurgical procedures or incorporate also other additional modules [38, 41, 42].

4.5. Interventional cardiology and cardiothoracic surgery

ANGIO Mentor™ (*3D Systems, formerly Simbionix*): it provides a virtual field created from CT/MRI images of real patients and data from cardiac intervention procedures (balloon angioplasty, coronary stenting). Standard guidewires, catheters, balloons, stents, and similar devices are used with the system. Monitoring the patient's vital signs and electrocardiographic changes is available. *ANGIO Mentor™* is a robust simulator used in many endovascular procedures, such as carotid stenting and renal, iliac, and other vascular interventions [43].

Vascular Intervention Simulation Trainer® (*VIST®, Mentice*): it is similar to the *ANGIO Mentor™* containing a library of virtual patients, tools, and procedures. These support tactile feedback and generate fluoroscopic images. It also supports a variety of other endovascular procedures, along with an electrophysiology module for training in pacemaker lead placement [43].

Vimedix™ (*CAE Healthcare*): it is an AR system for training in echocardiography. It consists of a mannequin and a transducer transthoracic or transesophageal echocardiogram. It has displayed face validity. Recently, *CAE Healthcare* has equipped it with *Hololens* in order to provide the ability to view the images with glasses, unrestricted from the dimensions of the screen [13]. *EchoCom* is another echocardiography AR trainer but for neonates. It has shown face, content, and construct validity [13].

Nakao Cardiac Model is a VR simulator for training in surgical palpitation of the beating heart. It supports haptic interaction. It does not include metrics tools and does not offer variability. The *Minimally Invasive Cardiac Surgery Simulator* by Berlage and colleagues is another VR simulator that virtually projects beating heart, ribs, and chest surface based on the patient's unique CT images. It is not interactive but supports variability of the simulated environments. A VR Lobectomy Simulator was developed by Solomon and colleagues. It includes video-assisted thoracoscopic surgery resection, lobectomy; it is controlled with haptic stimuli, and it has incorporated metrics tools that track performance, measure surgical times and errors, and ask questions [44].

dVSS™: cardiothoracic surgery also employs VR robotic training. A study found that the group previously trained in *dVSS™* performed better in robotic internal thoracic artery harvest and mitral valve annuloplasty than the control group [45].

4.6. Urology

URO Mentor™ (*3D Systems, formerly Simbionix*): a VR simulator for training in many urologic fields. It has shown educational benefit in cystoscopy and ureteroscopy [46]. It also supports several other modules, including essential skills, stone extraction, stone lithotripsy, cutting strictures, and taking biopsy modules. Face and content validity have been confirmed, and it is considered as a realistic and useful training model for endourological procedures.

University of Washington TURP Trainer (*University of Washington*): this VR trainer was designed for training in transurethral resection of the prostate (TURP). It has been extensively validated and shown face and construct validity. This is the only model to have shown concurrent validity with other assessment tools in studies with large numbers of participants [47, 48].

UROSim™ (*VirtaMed*): a commercial TURP VR simulator that has recurrently shown face, content, and construct validity. It simulates endoscopic movement and allows users to perform resection, coagulation, and also complete TURP operations. It can be adjusted to different levels of difficulty and has advanced metrics tools [47, 48].

Other TURP simulators using VR are the *PelvicVisionTURP simulator*, the *GreenLight laser simulator* (*GreenLight SIM, American Medical Systems Inc.*), and the *Kansai HoLEP simulator*. All these demonstrate face and construct validity [47, 48].

A module employing *Phantom® haptics interface* (*Geomagic*) was developed for digital rectal examination. However further research is required. The University of Grenoble developed in 2013 a VR simulator for transrectal ultrasound-guided prostate biopsy. Since then, several systems have been constructed [10]. Moreover, the *ProMIS®* laparoscopic VR trainer has displayed construct validity in urologic procedures [49]. Studies have compared the educational effect of VR trainers with that of bench models and found no difference in the early steps. However, VR trainers are far more expensive than bench models but also offer greater diversity [50]. AR has limited applications in urology training, as it is only used to teach theoretically the procedural steps. A relevant application based on *Google Glass* trains urology residents in how to place an inflatable penile prosthesis [51].

4.7. Orthopedics

The *ImmersiveTouch®* simulator is used in a variety of spine surgery procedures, including thoracic pedicle screw placement and percutaneous spinal needle placement. *Phantom®* haptics interface is used for spinal needle insertion. *Gaumard HAL S2001® and HAL S3000®* Mannequins and *Novint Falcon®* (*Novint Technologies*) are systems for vertebroplasty simulation training. A model from *Medtronic* has also been used in pedicle screw placement and placement of lateral mass screws [52].

Three VR models are validated and commercially available for training in arthroscopy. Both *Arthro MENTOR™ (3D Systems, formerly Simbionix*) which was the evolution of *ARTHRO-VR®*

(*GMV*) and *ArthroSIM* have displayed face, content, and construct validity [53–56]. *ArthroS™* (*Virtamed*) has demonstrated greater face validity than *Arthro MENTOR™* and *ArthroSIM* in a head-to-head comparison study [54].

4.8. Endovascular surgery

Usually, endovascular VR trainers have metric tools that evaluate the procedural time, the volume of the contrast used, and the time for fluoroscopy. They provide plenty of modules including angioplasty and stenting of coronary, renal, iliac, and femoral vessels. They also seem to benefit the inexperienced users, and the skills acquired seem to be transferable [57].

ANGIO Mentor™ (*3D Systems, formerly Simbionix*): it contains 23 different endovascular procedures and over 150 patient scenarios. It simulates the environment of endovascular procedures performed under fluoroscopy in the cath lab, interventional suite, or operating room. It supports haptic feedback, and it can benefit trainees of different disciplines, including interventional cardiology, interventional radiology, vascular surgery, electrophysiology, neuro surgery, and interventional neuroradiology and trauma. It has shown better procedure time, fluoroscopy time, and contrast volume in many procedures, such as carotid artery stenting, renal artery stenting, and cerebral artery angioplasty [42, 58].

Vascular Intervention Simulation Trainer® (*VIST®*, *Mentice*): as already mentioned it contains many training modules. It also supports haptic feedback and has many difficulty levels. Studies have shown improvement of users' performance in many endovascular procedures, including carotid artery, cerebral artery, renal artery, iliofemoral artery, aorta, and superficial femoral artery procedures [42, 58].

Cardio CT (*Shina System*), *SimSuite* (*Medical Simulation Corporation*), and the newer *Compass™ 2* (*Medical Simulation Corporation*) are other VR simulators that have not been so extensively studied [58].

4.9. Obstetrics and gynecology

HystSim™ and the newer *EssureSim™* (*both by VirtaMed*) are VR simulators for training in hysteroscopic procedures. Studies have attributed face, construct, and predictive validity to them and have also shown that the skills taught are retained for at least 2 weeks [59, 60]. A model from *CAE Healthcare* (the old *AccuTouch, Immersion*) has been used in hysteroscopy training and has shown construct validity and the ability to improve performance equally with box trainers [59].

MIST-VR might be suitable for training in gynecology training, as it has shown positive results in other fields [22]. *LapSim™* has also been used in salpingectomy training and shown construct validity [61]. AR has nonsignificant applications in gynecology training.

4.10. ENT

OtoSim™ (*OtoSim Inc.*): it is used in otoscopy training, offering a wide range of realistic images of the tympanic membrane and of various middle ear lesions. It was found to have good face validity [62].

VOXEL-MAN surgical simulator (*Hamburg, Germany*): it is a computer-based interface that can be used for temporal bone drilling and mastoidectomy. It supports *Phantom*® haptic devices for tactile feedback and 3D visual interfaces. It has demonstrated face, content, and construct validity [62–64]. Other similar simulators that display validity are the *Ohio State University surgical simulator*, the *Stanford Surgical Simulator* (*Stanford BioRobotics lab*), and the *Mediseus surgical simulator* (*CSIRO/University of Melbourne Temporal Bone Simulator*) [62–64].

Endoscopic Sinus Surgery Simulator (*ES3, Lockheed Martin*): it is used in sinus surgery, enabling haptic feedback with *Phantom*®. It collects and analyzes performance data providing performance metrics. It consists of three components: a workstation simulation platform (*Silicon Graphics Inc.*), a haptic controller, and an electromechanical human interaction platform with replica of an endoscope, surgical tools, and a mannequin. It is among the most widely validated sinus simulators, demonstrating content, concurrent, construct, and predictive validity and a significant retention of the acquired skills [62, 64]. *Dextroscope*® is also used in sinus surgery and has shown predictive validity [64].

dVSS™ is also used in robotic ENT surgery training. Tonsillectomy, fine-needle biopsy of the thyroid, myringotomy, nasal endoscopy, and cricothyroidotomy VR simulators have also been developed [62, 65].

4.11. Ophthalmology

Cataract and vitreoretinal surgery is the main field of VR training in ophthalmology. *EyeSi*® *simulator* (*VRmagic*) is the most commonly used system. It includes two pedals (one for the microscope and one for phacoemulsification/vitrectomy/infusion and aspiration modes), a physical head and eye, and a microscope, all connected to a computer. It does not support tactile feedback. However, it demonstrates construct and predictive validity. The educational effect is restricted to novices [66–68]. *MicrovisTouch*™ (*ImmersiveTouch*) and *PhacoVision*® (*Melerit Medical*) are additional models with only the *MicrovisTouch*™ supporting haptic feedback [66]. AR is still of limited use, although a study finds educational benefit when AR is applied in ophthalmoscopy teaching [69].

4.12. Other fields

Pediatrics and emergency medicine are promising fields for integration of VR training. Rigorous work is being done to create realistic virtual humans and virtual pediatric models. Moreover, highly realistic virtual environments that recreate massive destruction situations are being developed for use in emergency medicine [70, 71].

AR has been used in intubation training. More modern systems, such as *BRONCH Mentor*™ (*3D Systems, formerly Simbionix*) and *EndoVR Simulator*™, include intubation modules and have shown positive educational effect [72].

Ultrasonography simulators have been used for assessing trainees. *ScanTrainer*® (*MedaPhor*). It consists of a haptic force-feedback-enabled device and a computer with a touchscreen that visualizes ultrasonography images according to the user's movements [73].

EndoVR Simulator™, *BRONCH Mentor*™, and *ORSIM*® (*Airway Simulation Limited*) are some of the systems used for training in bronchoscopy [62]. Most of them have shown positive learning effects. *BRONCH Mentor*™ offers a bigger variety of pathologies and clinical situations and a more realistic environment. *ORSIM*® is a small, portable simulator with a physical bronchoscope and an interface based on regular laptops [74].

Some AR applications that indicate the landmarks for central venous catheterization have been developed. An ultrasound probe locates the vein and a microprojector projects it onto the skin. A study has found positive learning effect, when used in landmark finding training [75].

5. Conclusion and future perspectives

Most of the educational applications of VR and AR seem to have construct and predictive validity, with the acquired skills to be transferable to real situations. However, the credibility of several of these studied might be questionable. First of all, many of them are not randomized studies, with cohorts of different characteristics and inadequate number of participants (less than 30 in most studies). Moreover, there are few studies for each simulator, and there are no similar standards in their design, so that they could be summarized and directly compared. In addition, many of the studies referring to specific simulators become quickly outdated as they do not take into account the simulators' continuous upgrades. More randomized control trials, comparing the effect of VR training against no training, other simulation-based training, or different VR training systems, are needed. The samples must be larger to strengthen the results and the designs of different studies similar [5, 7, 8, 21]. Moreover, the extent of the decay of the skills over time must be elucidated. When these properties, along with the cost factors, are clarified, then we can examine the way that VR and AR can be officially incorporated in medical education curricula.

However, the published literature suggests a positive educational impact. VR/AR training displays certain advantages toward other simulation techniques. Although expensive to buy, VR/AR simulators provide a relatively costless opportunity for reproducible training under various environments and difficulty levels. Moreover, they do not raise ethical issues, compared with other animal and living tissue simulation models. They provide immersion for the user and the ability to perform complete procedures, in contrast with partial task trainers. Multiple studies have shown a favorable impact of VR/AR trainers on inexperienced trainees, and we can intuitively assume that they are technically evolving in high pace as the technology progresses. Future improvements could include the integration of olfactory stimuli. Odors can be used as diagnostic tools or even to recreate stressful conditions (e.g., in a combat or in the operating room) with greater realism [1, 8]. Medical informatics is also an evolving field. Medical data will be visualized more clearly and impressively with VR/AR technology. Users will be able to dive into statistical plots and reports, watch them in 4D (in 3D space and time), manipulate them, and "wander" around them. Although significant progress has been made, there is still a need for more processing power, higher resolution, better design of the scenarios, and more advanced haptic devices in order to achieve highly realistic environments [31, 76].

Author details

Panteleimon Pantelidis[1]*, Angeliki Chorti[1], Ioanna Papagiouvanni[1], Georgios Paparoidamis[1], Christos Drosos[1], Thrasyvoulos Panagiotakopoulos[1], Georgios Lales[1] and Michail Sideris[2]

*Address all correspondence to: pan.pantelidis@outlook.com

1 Aristotle University of Thessaloniki, Thessaloniki, Greece

2 Queen Mary University London (QMUL), London, UK

References

[1] Beolchi L, Riva G. Virtual reality for health care. In: Akay M, Marsh A, editors. Information Technologies in Medicine. Vol. 2. New York, USA: John Wiley & Sons, Inc.; 2001. pp. 39-83. DOI: 10.1002/0471206458.ch3

[2] Graur F. Virtual reality in medicine — Going beyond the limits. In: Sik-Lanyi C, editor. Thousand Faces Virtual Real. Rijeka, Croatia: InTech; 2014. pp. 23-35. DOI: 10.5772/59277

[3] Satava RM. Virtual reality surgical simulator. Surgical Endoscopy. 1993;**7**:203-205

[4] Langreth R. Virtual reality: Head mounted distress. Popular Science. 1994;**5**:49

[5] Vozenilek J. See one, do one, teach one: Advanced technology in medical education. Academic Emergency Medicine. 2004;**11**:1149-1154. DOI: 10.1197/j.aem.2004.08.003

[6] Riva G. Applications of virtual environments in medicine. Methods of Information in Medicine. 2003;**42**:524-534

[7] Kamphuis C, Barsom E, Schijven M, Christoph N. Augmented reality in medical education? Perspectives on Medical Education. 2014;**3**:300-311. DOI: 10.1007/s40037-013-0107-7

[8] Sakakushev BE, Marinov BI, Stefanova PP, Kostianev SS, Georgiou EK. Striving for better medical education: The simulation approach. Folia Medica (Plovdiv). 2017;**59**:123-131 DOI: 10.1515/folmed-2017-0039

[9] Hodges LF, Kooper R, Meyer TC, Rothbaum BO, Opdyke D, de Graaff JJ, et al. Virtual environments for treating the fear of heights. Computer. 1995;**28**:27-34. DOI: 10.1109/2.391038

[10] Hamacher A, Kim SJ, Cho ST, Pardeshi S, Lee SH, Eun S-J, et al. Application of virtual, augmented, and mixed reality to urology. International Neurourology Journal. 2016; **20**:172-181. DOI: 10.5213/inj.1632714.357

[11] ISO 9241-210:2010. Ergonomics of human-system interaction – Part 210: Human-centred design for interactive systems. Available from: https://www.iso.org/standard/52075.html

[12] Persson J. A review of the design and development processes of simulation for training in healthcare – A technology-centered versus a human-centered perspective. Applied Ergonomics. 2017;**58**:314-326. DOI: 10.1016/j.apergo.2016.07.007

[13] Barsom EZ, Graafland M, Schijven MP. Systematic review on the effectiveness of augmented reality applications in medical training. Surgical Endoscopy. 2016;**30**:4174-4183. DOI: 10.1007/s00464-016-4800-6

[14] Wang LL, Wu H-H, Bilici N, Tenney-Soeiro R. Gunner goggles: Implementing augmented reality into medical education. Studies in Health Technology and Informatics. 2016;**220**:446-449

[15] Albrecht U-V, Noll C, von Jan U. Explore and experience: Mobile augmented reality for medical training. Studies in Health Technology and Informatics. 2013;**192**:382-386

[16] Trelease RB. Anatomical informatics: Millennial perspectives on a newer frontier. The Anatomical Record. 2002;**269**:224-235. DOI: 10.1002/ar.10177

[17] Evans CH, Schenarts KD. Evolving educational techniques in surgical training. The Surgical Clinics of North America. 2016;**96**:71-88. DOI: 10.1016/j.suc.2015.09.005

[18] Badash I, Burtt K, Solorzano CA, Carey JN. Innovations in surgery simulation: A review of past, current and future techniques. Annals of Translational Medicine. 2016;**4**:453-453. DOI: 10.21037/atm.2016.12.24

[19] Paschold M, Huber T, Zeißig SR, Lang H, Kneist W. Tailored instructor feedback leads to more effective virtual-reality laparoscopic training. Surgical Endoscopy. 2014;**28**: 967-973. DOI: 10.1007/s00464-013-3258-z

[20] Larsen CR, Oestergaard J, Ottesen BS, Soerensen JL. The efficacy of virtual reality simulation training in laparoscopy: A systematic review of randomized trials: Virtual reality simulation: A review. Acta Obstetricia et Gynecologica Scandinavica. 2012;**91**:1015-1028. DOI: 10.1111/j.1600-0412.2012.01482.x

[21] Beyer-Berjot L, Aggarwal R. Toward technology-supported surgical training: The potential of virtual simulators in laparoscopic surgery. Scandinavian Journal of Surgery. 2013;**102**:221-226. DOI: 10.1177/1457496913496494

[22] Hammond I, Karthigasu K. Training, assessment and competency in gynaecologic surgery. Best Practice & Research. Clinical Obstetrics & Gynaecology. 2006;**20**:173-187. DOI: 10.1016/j.bpobgyn.2005.09.006

[23] Cole SJ, Mackenzie H, Ha J, Hanna GB, Miskovic D. Randomized controlled trial on the effect of coaching in simulated laparoscopic training. Surgical Endoscopy. 2014;**28**: 979-986. DOI: 10.1007/s00464-013-3265-0

[24] Khan MW, Lin D, Marlow N, Altree M, Babidge W, Field J, et al. Laparoscopic skills maintenance: A randomized trial of virtual reality and box trainer simulators. Journal of Surgical Education. 2014;**71**:79-84. DOI: 10.1016/j.jsurg.2013.05.009

[25] Vera AM, Russo M, Mohsin A, Tsuda S. Augmented reality telementoring (ART) platform: A randomized controlled trial to assess the efficacy of a new surgical education technology. Surgical Endoscopy. 2014;**28**:3467-3472. DOI: 10.1007/s00464-014-3625-4

[26] Dixon BJ, Daly MJ, Chan HHL, Vescan A, Witterick IJ, Irish JC. Inattentional blindness increased with augmented reality surgical navigation. American Journal of Rhinology & Allergy. 2014;**28**:433-437. DOI: 10.2500/ajra.2014.28.4067

[27] Lallas CD. Davis and Members of the society of JW. Robotic surgery training with commercially available simulation systems in 2011: A current review and practice pattern survey from the society of urologic robotic surgeons. Journal of Endourology. 2012;**26**:283-293. DOI: 10.1089/end.2011.0371

[28] Kiely DJ, Gotlieb WH, Lau S, Zeng X, Samouelian V, Ramanakumar AV, et al. Virtual reality robotic surgery simulation curriculum to teach robotic suturing: A randomized controlled trial. Journal of Robotic Surgery. 2015;**9**:179-186. DOI: 10.1007/s11701-015-0513-4

[29] Vaccaro CM, Crisp CC, Fellner AN, Jackson C, Kleeman SD, Pavelka J. Robotic virtual reality simulation plus standard robotic orientation versus standard robotic orientation alone: A randomized controlled trial. Female Pelvic Medicine & Reconstructive Surgery. 2013;**19**:266-270. DOI: 10.1097/SPV.0b013e3182a09101

[30] Liu M, Curet M. A review of training research and virtual reality simulators for the da Vinci surgical system. Teaching and Learning in Medicine. 2015;**27**:12-26. DOI: 10.1080/10401334.2014.979181

[31] Davies J, Khatib M, Bello F. Open surgical simulation—A review. Journal of Surgical Education. 2013;**70**:618-627. DOI: 10.1016/j.jsurg.2013.04.007

[32] van der Wiel SE, Küttner Magalhães R, Rocha Gonçalves CR, Dinis-Ribeiro M, Bruno MJ, Koch AD. Simulator training in gastrointestinal endoscopy – From basic training to advanced endoscopic procedures. Best Practice & Research. Clinical Gastroenterology. 2016;**30**:375-387. DOI: 10.1016/j.bpg.2016.04.004

[33] Harpham-Lockyer L. Role of virtual reality simulation in endoscopy training. World Journal of Gastrointestinal Endoscopy. 2015;**7**:1287. DOI: 10.4253/wjge.v7.i18.1287

[34] Hashimoto DA, Petrusa E, Phitayakorn R, Valle C, Casey B, Gee D. A proficiency-based virtual reality endoscopy curriculum improves performance on the fundamentals of endoscopic surgery examination. Surgical Endoscopy. DOI: 10.1007/s00464-017-5821-5

[35] Ekkelenkamp VE, Koch AD, de Man RA, Kuipers EJ. Training and competence assessment in GI endoscopy: A systematic review. Gut. 2016;**65**:607-615. DOI: 10.1136/gutjnl-2014-307173

[36] Pelargos PE, Nagasawa DT, Lagman C, Tenn S, Demos JV, Lee SJ, et al. Utilizing virtual and augmented reality for educational and clinical enhancements in neurosurgery. Journal of Clinical Neuroscience. 2017;**35**:1-4. DOI: 10.1016/j.jocn.2016.09.002

[37] Konakondla S, Fong R, Schirmer CM. Simulation training in neurosurgery: Advances in education and practice. Advances in Medical Education and Practice. 2017;**8**:465-473. DOI: 10.2147/AMEP.S113565

[38] Rehder R, Abd-El-Barr M, Hooten K, Weinstock P, Madsen JR, Cohen AR. The role of simulation in neurosurgery. Child's Nervous System. 2016;**32**:43-54. DOI: 10.1007/s00381-015-2923-z

[39] Yudkowsky R, Luciano C, Banerjee P, Schwartz A, Alaraj A, Lemole GMJ, et al. Practice on an augmented reality/haptic simulator and library of virtual brains improves residents' ability to perform a ventriculostomy. Simulation in Healthcare: The Journal of the Society for Simulation in Healthcare. 2013;**8**:25-31. DOI: 10.1097/SIH.0b013e3182662c69

[40] Alaraj A, Charbel FT, Birk D, Tobin M, Luciano C, Banerjee PP, et al. Role of cranial and spinal virtual and augmented reality simulation using immersive touch modules in neurosurgical training. Neurosurgery. 2013;**72**(Suppl 1):115-123. DOI: 10.1227/NEU.0b013e3182753093

[41] Kirkman MA, Ahmed M, Albert AF, Wilson MH, Nandi D, Sevdalis N. The use of simulation in neurosurgical education and training: A systematic review. Journal of Neurosurgery. 2014;**121**:228-246. DOI: 10.3171/2014.5.JNS131766

[42] Mitha AP, Almekhlafi MA, Janjua MJJ, Albuquerque FC, McDougall CG. Simulation and augmented reality in endovascular neurosurgery: Lessons from aviation. Neurosurgery. 2013;**72**(Suppl 1):107-114. DOI: 10.1227/NEU.0b013e31827981fd

[43] Lake CL. Simulation in cardiology and cardiothoracic and vascular surgery. Seminars in Cardiothoracic and Vascular Anesthesia. 2005;**9**:325-333-1. DOI: 10.1177/108925320500900405

[44] Trehan K, Kemp CD, Yang SC. Simulation in cardiothoracic surgical training: Where do we stand? The Journal of Thoracic and Cardiovascular Surgery. 2014;**147**:18-24.e2. DOI: 10.1016/j.jtcvs.2013.09.007

[45] Valdis M, Chu MWA, Schlachta CM, Kiaii B. Validation of a novel virtual reality training curriculum for robotic cardiac surgery: A randomized trial. Innovations: Technology and Techniques in Cardiothoracic and Vascular Surgery. 2015;**10**:383-388. DOI: 10.1097/IMI.0000000000000222

[46] Watterson JD, Beiko DT, Kuan JK, Denstedt JD. Randomized prospective blinded study validating acquisition of ureteroscopy skills using computer based virtual reality endourological simulator. The Journal of Urology. 2002;**168**:1928-1932. DOI: 10.1097/01.ju.0000034357.84449.56

[47] Viswaroop SB, Gopalakrishnan G, Kandasami SV. Role of transurethral resection of the prostate simulators for training in transurethral surgery. Current Opinion in Urology. 2015;**25**:153-157. DOI: 10.1097/MOU.0000000000000141

[48] Khan R, Aydin A, Khan MS, Dasgupta P, Ahmed K. Simulation-based training for prostate surgery. BJU International. 2015;**116**:665-674. DOI: 10.1111/bju.12721

[49] Feifer A, Delisle J, Anidjar M. Hybrid augmented reality simulator: Preliminary construct validation of laparoscopic smoothness in a urology residency program. The Journal of Urology. 2008;**180**:1455-1459. DOI: 10.1016/j.juro.2008.06.042

[50] Chou DS, Abdelshehid C, Clayman RV, McDougall EM. Comparison of results of virtual-reality simulator and training model for basic Ureteroscopy training. Journal of Endourology. 2006;**20**:266-271. DOI: 10.1089/end.2006.20.266

[51] Dickey RM, Srikishen N, Lipshultz LI, Spiess PE, Carrion RE, Hakky TS. Augmented reality assisted surgery: A urologic training tool. Asian Journal of Andrology. 2016;**18**: 732-734. DOI: 10.4103/1008-682X.166436

[52] Pfandler M, Lazarovici M, Stefan P, Wucherer P, Weigl M. Virtual reality-based simulators for spine surgery: A systematic review. The Spine Journal. 2017;**17**:1352-63. DOI: 10.1016/j.spinee.2017.05.016

[53] LeBel M-E, Haverstock J, Cristancho S, van Eimeren L, Buckingham G. Observational learning during simulation-based training in arthroscopy: Is it useful to novices? Journal of Surgical Education. DOI: 10.1016/j.jsurg.2017.06.005

[54] Martin KD, Akoh CC, Amendola A, Phisitkul P. Comparison of three virtual reality arthroscopic simulators as part of an orthopedic residency educational curriculum. The Iowa Orthopaedic Journal. 2016;**36**:20-25

[55] Bayona S, Fernández-Arroyo JM, Martín I, Bayona P. Assessment study of insight ARTHRO VR® arthroscopy virtual training simulator: Face, content, and construct validities. Journal of Robotic Surgery. 2008;**2**:151-158. DOI: 10.1007/s11701-008-0101-y

[56] Obdeijn MC, Bavinck N, Mathoulin C, van der Horst CMAM, Schijven MP, Tuijthof GJM. Education in wrist arthroscopy: Past, present and future. Knee Surgery, Sports Traumatology, Arthroscopy. 2015;**23**:1337-1345. DOI: 10.1007/s00167-013-2592-y

[57] Tsang JS, Naughton PA, Leong S, Hill ADK, Kelly CJ, Leahy AL. Virtual reality simulation in endovascular surgical training. Surgeon. 2008;**6**:214-220

[58] See KWM, Chui KH, Chan WH, Wong KC, Chan YC. Evidence for endovascular simulation training: A systematic review. European Journal of Vascular and Endovascular Surgery. 2016;**51**:441-451. DOI: 10.1016/j.ejvs.2015.10.011

[59] Savran MM, Sørensen SMD, Konge L, Tolsgaard MG, Bjerrum F. Training and assessment of hysteroscopic skills: A systematic review. Journal of Surgical Education. 2016; **73**:906-918. DOI: 10.1016/j.jsurg.2016.04.006

[60] Janse JA, Goedegebuure RSA, Veersema S, Broekmans FJM, Schreuder HWR. Hysteroscopic sterilization using a virtual reality simulator: Assessment of learning curve. Journal of Minimally Invasive Gynecology. 2013;**20**:775-782. DOI: 10.1016/j.jmig.2013.04.016

[61] Aggarwal R, Tully A, Grantcharov T, Larsen C, Miskry T, Farthing A, et al. Virtual reality simulation training can improve technical skills during laparoscopic salpingectomy for ectopic pregnancy. BJOG: An International Journal of Obstetrics & Gynaecology. 2006;**113**:1382-1387. DOI: 10.1111/j.1471-0528.2006.01148.x

[62] Javia L, Sardesai MG. Physical models and virtual reality simulators in otolaryngology. Otolaryngologic Clinics of North America. 2017;**50**:875-891. DOI: 10.1016/j.otc.2017.05.001

[63] Andersen SAW. Virtual reality simulation training of mastoidectomy – Studies on novice performance. Danish Medical Journal. 2016;**63**:B5277

[64] Arora A, Lau LYM, Awad Z, Darzi A, Singh A, Tolley N. Virtual reality simulation training in otolaryngology. International Journal of Surgery. 2014;**12**:87-94. DOI: 10.1016/j.ijsu.2013.11.007

[65] Burns JA, Adkins LK, Dailey S, Klein AM. Simulators for laryngeal and airway surgery. Otolaryngologic Clinics of North America. 2017;**50**:903-922. DOI: 10.1016/j.otc.2017.05.003

[66] Sikder S, Tuwairqi K, Al-Kahtani E, Myers WG, Banerjee P. Surgical simulators in cataract surgery training. The British Journal of Ophthalmology. 2014;**98**:154-158. DOI: 10.1136/bjophthalmol-2013-303700

[67] Thomsen ASS, Bach-Holm D, Kjærbo H, Højgaard-Olsen K, Subhi Y, Saleh GM, et al. Operating room performance improves after proficiency-based virtual reality cataract surgery training. Ophthalmology. 2017;**124**:524-531. DOI: 10.1016/j.ophtha.2016.11.015

[68] Gillan SN, Saleh GM. Ophthalmic surgical simulation: A new era. JAMA Ophthalmology. 2013;**131**:1623. DOI: 10.1001/jamaophthalmol.2013.1011

[69] Leitritz MA, Ziemssen F, Suesskind D, Partsch M, Voykov B, Bartz-Schmidt KU, et al. Critical evaluation of the usability of augmented reality ophthalmoscopy for the training of inexperienced examiners. Retina (Phila, PA). 2014;**34**:785-791. DOI: 10.1097/IAE.0b013e3182a2e75d

[70] Lopreiato JO, Sawyer T. Simulation-based medical education in pediatrics. Academic Pediatrics. 2015;**15**:134-142. DOI: 10.1016/j.acap.2014.10.010

[71] Reznek M, Harter P, Krummel T. Virtual reality and simulation: Training the future emergency physician. Academic Emergency Medicine: Official Journal of the Society for Academic Emergency Medicine. 2002;**9**:78-87

[72] Nilsson PM, Russell L, Ringsted C, Hertz P, Konge L. Simulation-based training in flexible fibreoptic intubation: A randomised study. European Journal of Anaesthesiology. 2015;**32**:609-614. DOI: 10.1097/EJA.0000000000000092

[73] Jensen JK, Dyre L, Jørgensen ME, Andreasen LA, Tolsgaard MG. Collecting validity evidence for simulation-based assessment of point-of-care ultrasound skills: Simulation-based ultrasound assessment. Journal of Ultrasound in Medicine. 2017;**36**:2475-2483. DOI: 10.1002/jum.14292

[74] Naur TMH, Nilsson PM, Pietersen PI, Clementsen PF, Konge L. Simulation-based training in flexible bronchoscopy and Endobronchial ultrasound-guided Transbronchial needle aspiration (EBUS-TBNA): A systematic review. Respiration. 2017;**93**:355-362. DOI: 10.1159/000464331

[75] Jeon Y, Choi S, Kim H. Evaluation of a simplified augmented reality device for ultrasound-guided vascular access in a vascular phantom. Journal of Clinical Anesthesia. 2014;**26**:485-489. DOI: 10.1016/j.jclinane.2014.02.010

[76] Kapoor S. Haptics – Touchfeedback technology widening the horizon of medicine. Journal of Clinical and Diagnostic Research. 2014;**8**:294-299. DOI: 10.7860/JCDR/2014/7814.4191

Chapter 6

Proposed Synthetic Tissues that Replace Human Cadavers for Training

Emily Earl and Hadi Mohammadi

Additional information is available at the end of the chapter

http://dx.doi.org/10.5772/intechopen.73245

Abstract

In order to develop surgical skills required for cardiac surgeries, such as with surgeries of all types, years of practice and experience is required. Young cardiac surgeons need to improve technical proficiency in order to enrich the quality of care provided and to ensure patient safety. Realistic synthetic platforms and models are common resources for teaching and enhancing practical skills for both inexperienced as well as senior medical students, however are found particularly useful for young surgeons in training. Appropriate and available educational platforms can play an increasingly vital role in the training progression for young trainees in the area of cardiothoracic surgery. For example, the Coronary Artery Bypass Graft (CABG) surgery encompasses an extensive range of pathologic anatomies and surgical performances. In this chapter, we present original, synthetic, biomimetic models that allows for the accurate practice of surgeries such as the CABG surgery and aortic valve implantation. The prototype uses a polyvinyl alcohol (PVA) cryogel specifically designed to mimic the geometric properties of vasculature and the tissue of heart valve leaflets. The proposed models both visually resemble and feel like human tissue in addition to possessing relatively consistent mechanical properties. The technology and platform proposed have the potential for application in all cardiovascular-related reconstructive surgeries.

Keywords: hydrogel biomaterials, surgical tools, cardiac training, aortic valves, reconstructive surgery, bypass surgery, CABG

1. Introduction

The number of incidents of severe aortic stenosis in adults is remarkably high [1]. However, suitable timing of aortic valve replacement has the potential to avoid both early and late fatal events as well as result in improved functional status of the valve. Early diagnosis and treatment will lead to increased preservation of regular ventricular function in addition to the possibility of regaining regular ventricular function from previously irregularly functioning valves. As the basis for the decision to proceed with surgical interventions is how the regular function and structure of the left ventricle, aortic valve and ascending aorta can be affected by appropriately timed and performed valve replacements, it is crucial to understand the implications of these factors.

Aortic stenosis is typically a progressive disease and with increasing stenosis severity there is an increased resistance during left ventricular outflow. In order for the left ventricle to compensate this high resistance while still maintaining normal systemic pressure and cardiac output, a higher left ventricular pressure is generated. This elevated pressure is achieved by concentric ventricular hypertrophy, an increase of mass and thickness in the wall of the left ventricle. Although this might be an effective temporary solution, the left ventricle will eventually exceed the limit of concentric hypertrophy and begin to dilate in order to maintain left ventricular pump function. This dilation leads to a change in the shape of the left ventricle which may induce significant and negative affects to the valves function. Factors such as ejection fraction and fiber shortening suggest that velocity may eventually be reduced, leading to congestive heart failure.

Both phases, that is, cardiac hypertrophy and ventricular wall dilation, could have possible effects on both the hemodynamic and metabolic alternations. As the ventricular wall experiences progressive dilation and increased hypertrophy, the end-diastolic and pulmonary venous pressure increase may lead to an increase in shortness of breath. In addition, as the myocardial wall tension increases due to hypertrophy, more oxygen is required and because the supply of oxygen remains unchanged, myocardial ischemia and the symptom of angina pectoris may occur. Further, the alteration in ventricular shape and dynamics caused from excessive dilation of the left ventricle may create a vicious cycle, inducing chronic congestive heart failure.

Aortic valve replacement will provide a significant reduction of these symptoms and enhanced function for patients with ventricular dysfunction. Even in cases of congestive heart failure and noticeable ineffectiveness of ventricular function, aortic valve replacement may lead to improvement in symptoms and ventricular function, resulting in the reversibility of ventricular dysfunction and improved survival. Hemodynamic assessment of the valve stenosis involves the determination of the valvular gradient and an estimation of both the aortic valve area and the aortic valve area index. If the ejection fraction and cardiac output are normal, severe aortic stenosis is detected by a pressure gradient across the valve with a value equal to or greater than 50 mmHg or by an aortic valve area index that is less than 0.75 cm^2/m^2 [1]. If the cardiac output is lower than normal, opposed to the pressure gradient the valve area index must be considered as the pressure gradient across the valve can be minimal for decreased cardiac outflow. Aortic valve replacement is recommended even in the presence of a left ventricular ejection fraction that is less than 25% as well as for symptomatic patients with moderate aortic stenosis in which the aortic valve area is in the range of 0.7–1.2 cm^2 [1].

An artificial platform which can be used to simulate aortic heart valve replacement or coronary artery bypass surgery does not exist. Current possible options are based on synthetic models that lack adequate realism or animal models which are not available for repetitive practice. It should also be noted that there are multiple limitations in using animal models which do not occur with our proposed synthetic models.

In this study we design and develop synthetic models of ascending aorta which have similar mechanical properties and geometry to those of porcine tissue. The aortic valve, root and other sections, which are made all in one piece, bear physical resemblance to their counterparts of the porcine ascending aorta tissue. In addition to appearing similar to porcine tissue, our proposed models also feel like the tissue so that when sutures are performed it resembles a realistic platform as is experienced in an actual surgical operation. Additionally, we propose synthetic phantoms of coronary artery vascular grafts with objectively analogous geometrical properties. These phantoms also have reliable mechanical properties to that of the native tissue. The proposed platform is an outstanding tool which may be utilized for the simulation of anastomosis as implemented in coronary artery bypass surgery.

2. Method

2.1. Part A: aortic valve replacement surgery

In this study, the human ascending aorta made of cryogel-based biomaterials is proposed. To develop the geometry of the root, an innovative surfacing method related to the de Casteljau technique which is used for developing Bezier surfaces is implemented. The 3D geometry of this model is developed using 2D images attained from the axial dissection of a young adult porcine aortic root. The biomaterial implemented for the aortic valve is a blood-compatible cryogel made of polyvinyl alcohol (PVA-c) which is strengthened by bacterial cellulose (BC) natural nanofibers in a mixture of 15% PVA-c and 0.5% BC by weight fraction and the biomaterial implemented for the root is 10% PVA-c. The tensile properties of the fabricated PVA-BC were measured and are similar to those of the porcine aortic valve leaflet tissue in the two radial and circumferential directions. We also attained a near match of the stress-strain curves for the aorta in the circumferential and axial directions by applying 10% PVA-c with 75% initial strain after cycle 3 [2]. A cavity mold was designed and manufactured and the proposed polymeric valve was then fabricated. An extensive finite element analysis was performed in order to optimize the final product (please see the appendix). The proposed model may be further used for animal trials.

2.1.1. *Preparation of the hydrogel biomaterial*

Hydrolyzed PVA, 99+% (Sigma-Aldrich) with a molecular weight of 146,000–186,000 is used as the main ingredient for the solution preparation. A suspension of 0.877 wt% BC in distilled water is then added to the PVA solution. The BC solution is produced in shake flasks by a fermentation process using the *Acetobacter xylinum* bacterium. The BC suspension was prepared and added to the PVA solution. The new solution contains 15% PVA and 0.5% BC by weight fraction while the rest is distilled water as shown in **Figure 1** [3].

The final solution was dispensed into three metallic molds and placed in a heated/refrigerated circulator (15L Heating Bath Circulator Model SD15H170-A11B). The molds were cycled once between 20 and −20°C at 0.1°C/min for the solution to solidify and gain a deterministic shape (cycle 1). In order to impose anisotropy to the samples, a 75% strain was applied to all three

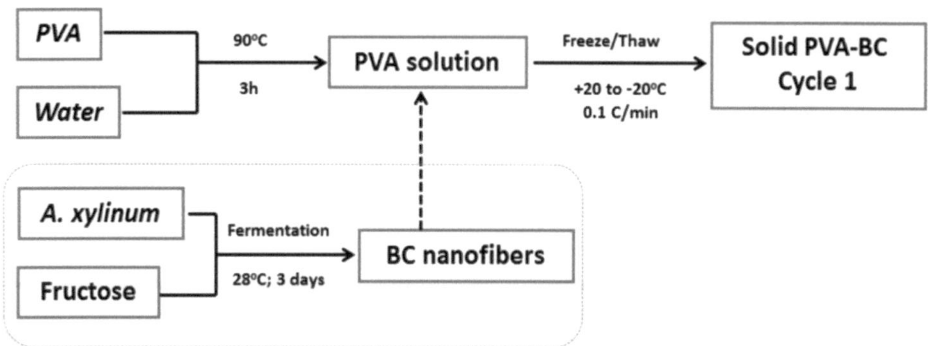

Figure 1. The proposed platform as to the PVA-BC nanocomposite preparation for the newly designed ascending aorta.

samples while they were placed back into the mold to reach the maximum anisotropy [3, 4]. The direction of stretch was selected to be in the direction with the higher stiffness, however one of the samples was kept non-stretched as a control. The molds were cycled using the freeze-thaw procedure for six cycles where one of the molds was removed at the end of each cycle. The above procedure and PVA-BC were applied for the preparation of the hydrogel implementation in the leaflet structure and a similar procedure was applied for the aortic wall, however as less stiffness is required for the aortic wall, BC fibers were not used and only 10% PVA was implemented.

2.1.2. Tensile testing

The results of the experimental tensile tests are reported in the form of load versus extension. These values are converted into stress-strain values by using the dimensions of the samples and the initial gauge length after preconditioning. Given that the samples undergo large deformation, the stress-strain curves obtained for all samples are nonlinear and hyperelastic. To fit the data obtained, an appropriate constitutive model is applied such that [2], $\sigma = y_0 + A\exp(B\varepsilon)$, where σ is true stress, ε is true strain and y_0, A, and B are constants.

The tensile properties are measured by a servohydraulic testing machine (INSTRON 8872) with a precise load cell that has a maximum capacity of 1 kg. In order to remain consistent with the realistic bio-environment of the samples, all measurements are carried out inside a container filled with distilled water at body temperature. The strain rate for the performed tensile tests is set to 40 mm/s with a maximum of 60% strain. The preconditioning test was achieved for all samples in 10 cycles with an amplitude of 5 cm and a frequency of 2 cycles/s [5, 6]. The mechanical properties obtained for the aortic valve and the ascending aorta are shown in **Figure 2a–d**. A close match in mechanical properties for the applied PVA-c samples and the porcine aorta was obtained. **Figure 2e** shows the stress-strain curves of the aorta in both principal directions and the anisotropic PVA-c sample after cycle 3 at 75% initial strain.

2.1.3. The design and fabrication of the ascending aorta

For the design of the geometry of both the ascending aorta and the aortic valve, an advanced and novel surfacing technique based on the de Casteljau method is applied on the Bezier-based

http://dx.doi.org/10.5772/intechopen.73245

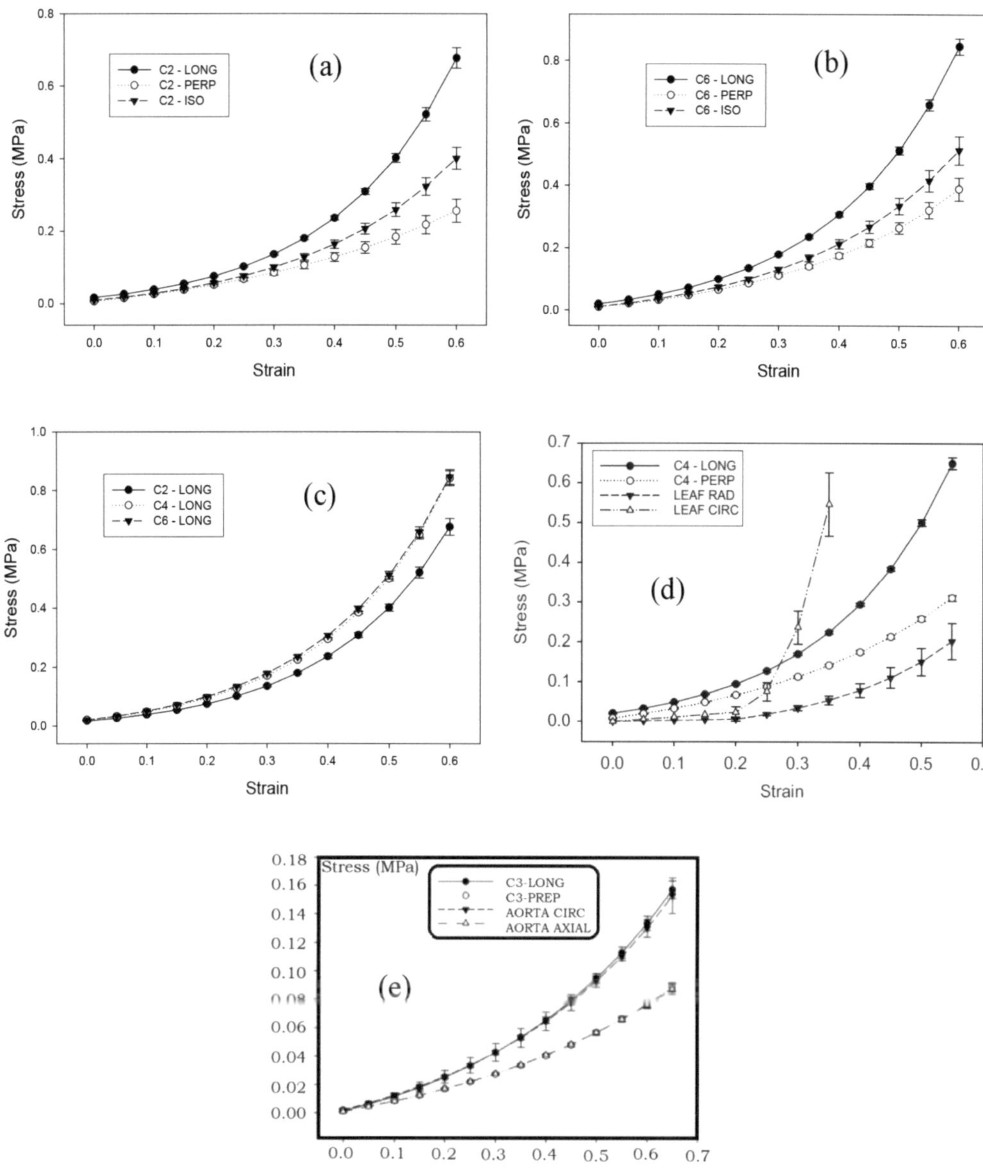

Figure 2. (a) The utilized anisotropy after cycle 2 at 75% initial strain, (b) the utilized anisotropy after cycle 6 at 75% initial strain, (c) the stress-strain curves in the longitudinal direction in cycle 2, 4 and 6 at 75% initial strain, (d) the tensile properties of the developed hydrogel [C4 is cycle 4, LONG stands for longitudinal, PERP stands for perpendicular, LEAF RAD stands for porcine aortic leaflet in the radial direction, LEAF CIRC stands for porcine aortic leaflet in the circumferential direction and the physiological domain represents the physiological loading condition of the valve] and (e) the closest match of the tensile stress-strain curves of aorta in both directions obtained from the anisotropic PVA at 75% initial strain after cycle 3 [6].

surfaces. The 3D geometry was developed by stacking 2D images obtained by the axial dissection of an adult human aortic root and aortic valve. It should be mentioned that the valve used for this purpose was a Mitroflow bioprosthetic valve. The 2D images are digitized and converted into a finite number of control points. This is determined by mapping the 2D geometry of each section using a coordinate measuring machine (CMM) with a laser scanning system such as 3D Digital Corp, 3D scanner cyberware.

The control points are then applied to construct the corresponding Bezier curves to complete the digitization of the 2D images which are used as the bases for the production of the final Bezier surfaces. The main advantage of this technique is that the final surface obtained is easily and quickly tunable. In order to increase the surface quality and apply any desired changes, Bezier curves are accustomed through a trial and error procedure by removing, relocating or interpolating the initial control points. The final surfaces are then brought to a CAD software environment by using a command as known as shell, for example, command Shell of I-Deas. As we are developing 3D and physical models, the thicknesses of the valve leaflets and ascending aortic wall and their respective variation is of particular importance. For this purpose, two surfaces are independently designed to form the top surfaces of both the male and female parts of the mold for each model. Even though the produced shells of the Bezier surfaces possess uniform thicknesses individually, the final products are 3D and have proper variable thicknesses as intended [6–8].

The thickness of the model is developed by the gap in the final design of the mold which is created due to the distance between these two surfaces. We used Mechanical Desktop V2013i CAD software for the perfection of the models throughout testing. As mentioned earlier, the geometry of the proposed aortic valve is inspired by a design modification on the Mitroflow bioprosthetic valve.

A major advantage of this new design is that the variable thickness of the leaflets is considered (0.7 mm on the free edge and 1.2 mm on the attachment with the stent) which is defined by applying a comprehensive finite element structural analysis and using the related optimized computational methods for further enhancement. The final model of the proposed valve consists of three identical cusps for which the leaflets are symmetrical about their own midlines. The fabricated model and the final prototype for the proposed aortic valve prosthesis composed of PBS thermoplastic material are shown in **Figure 3**. The valve is then added to the ascending aortic wall model to develop a complete synthetic model (made of PBS thermoplastic material) including the sinuses, two outlets for the right and left coronary arteries and the valve in only one component. The final model of the ascending aorta is shown in **Figure 4**.

2.1.4. Final models made of the proposed hydrogel

The developed material which possesses similar mechanical properties to those of the ascending aortic wall and the porcine heart valve leaflet tissue is implemented in the final models. The designed and fabricated molds were filled with the proposed hydrogels (PVA-BC for the valve leaflet and PVA only for the aortic wall) and the final models were manufactured. These models are similar in geometry and mechanical properties to that of the native tissues and can be an excellent tool for the simulation of aortic heart valve surgery (**Figure 5**).

The anatomy of the aortic valve is shown in **Figures 6** and **7**. **Figure 6** shows the valve from above, with the orientation as is usually seen throughout a standard transverse aortotomy [9].

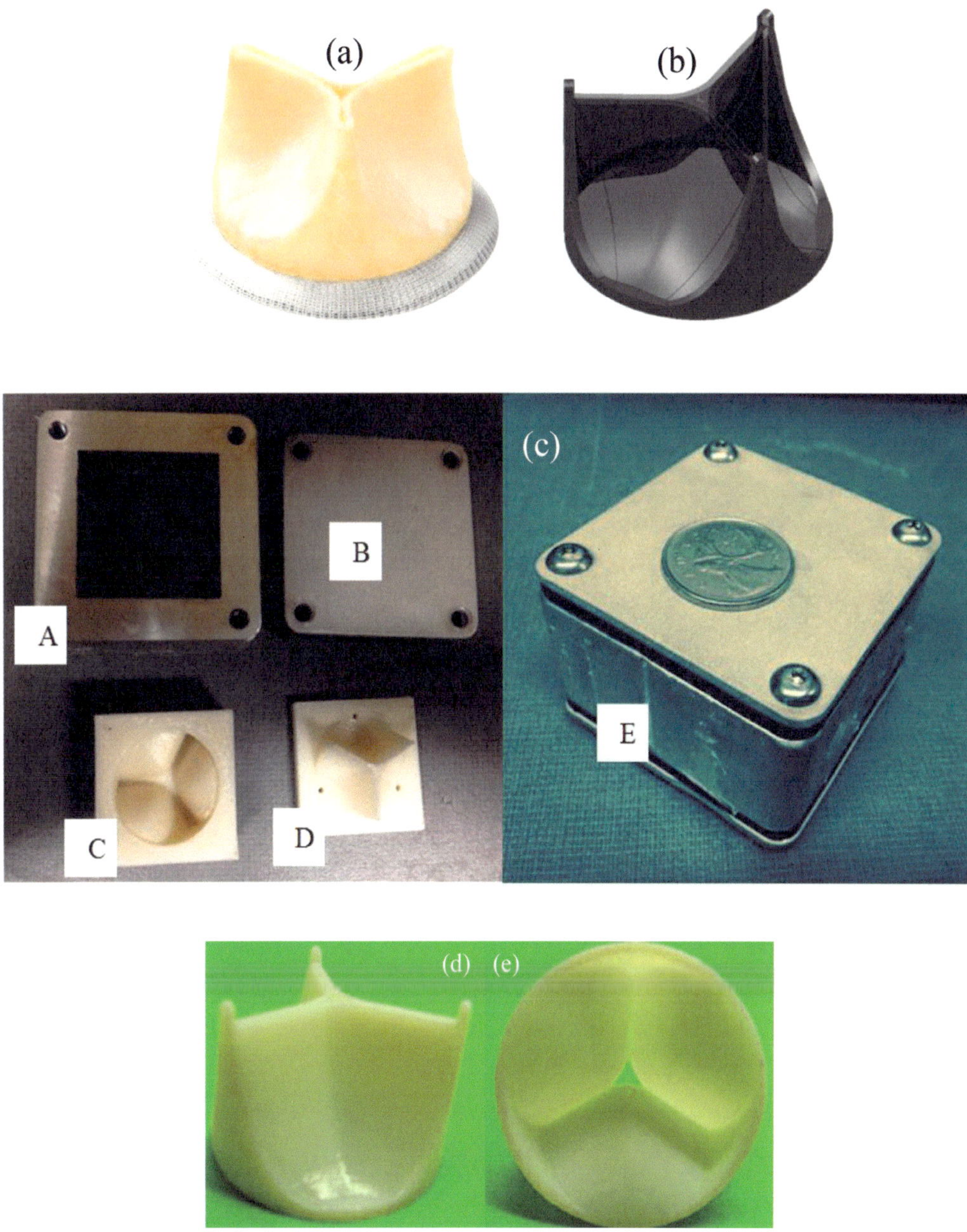

Figure 3. (a) The mitroflow bioprosthetic valve of which the design of the proposed valve is inspired, (b) the final CAD model of the proposed valve, (c) the designed and fabricated mold and its parts for the new design of the PVA-BC polymeric trileaflet valve. A: casing, B: caps ×2, C: main female part, D: main male part, E: the assembled mold, (d) and (e) are the first prototypes of the valve made of PBC thermoplastic material.

2.1.5. Surgical procedure

A transverse aortotomy is made which is normally placed approximately 15 mm above the level of the right coronary artery. This specific placement is to reduce the possibility of jeopardizing the

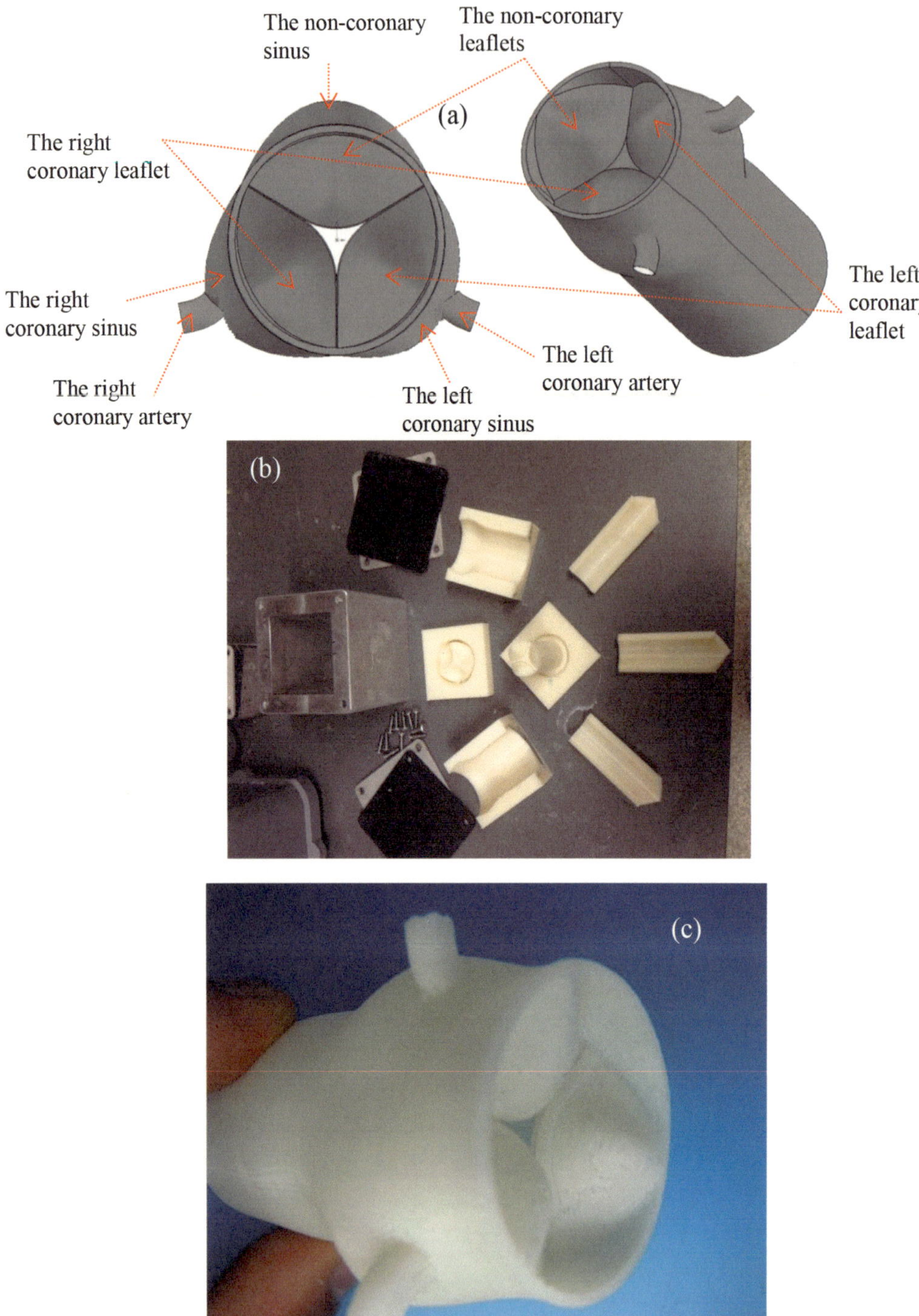

Figure 4. (a) The 3D CAD model of the ascending aorta, (b) the fabricated mold and its part of the proposed final CAD model, (c) the prototype of the ascending aorta made of PBC thermoplastic material including the left and right coronary arteries, the sinuses and the aortic valve in a singular component.

http://dx.doi.org/10.5772/intechopen.73245

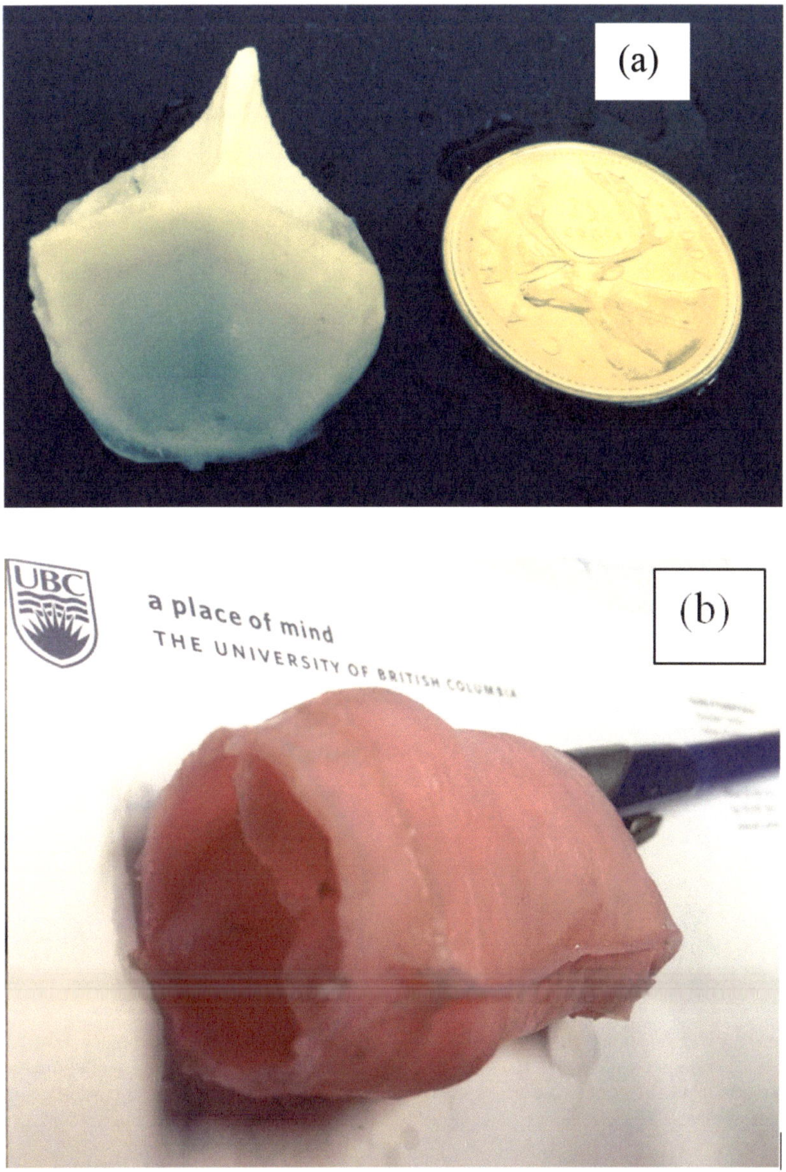

Figure 5. (a) The final aortic valve made of PVA-BC and (b) the final aortic root including the valve and sinuses with similar mechanical properties and geometry to that of the native tissue.

right coronary artery (caused by low incision placement) which can lead to technical complications in valve seating and aortotomy closure. Avoiding higher incision placement has decreased importance as the aortotomy can easily be angled downward and the anterior lip caused by a high incision can be quickly pulled back. The aortotomy is suggested to be extended to about 10 mm above the commissure between the left and right coronary leaflets and to a similar distance above the commissure between the left and the noncoronary leaflets [9].

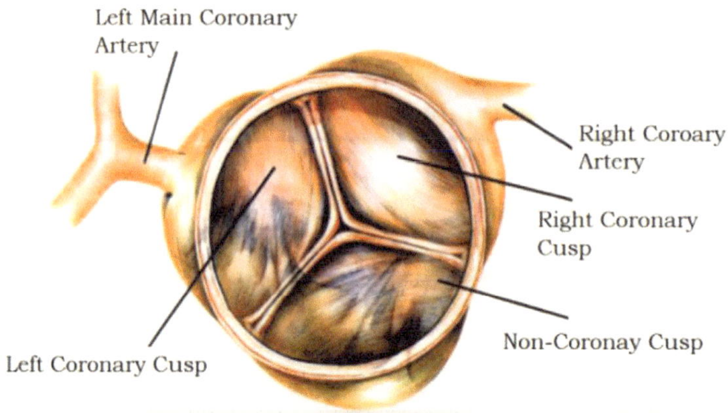

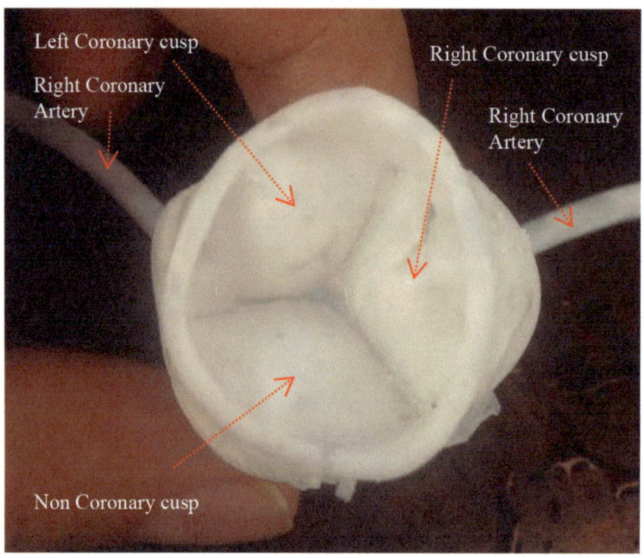

Figure 6. The anatomy of the human aortic valve including the right, left and noncoronary cusps (leaflets) as well as the main branches of left and right coronary arteries—top view. The top image is a typical diagram of the ascending aorta and the lower image is the synthetic ascending aorta proposed in this study which is one piece of the aortic root including the valve and coronary outlets.

After retractors are located, the valve can be seen, and the approach for excision is identified the calcified tissues are completely excised, ensuring to take care to not injure the bundle of His or the aortic wall. In many severely calcified valves, leaflets are free of calcification at the site of attachment prior to the annulus so the incision line can be positioned exactly on the calcium-free ribbon near the annulus. If a calcium-free ribbon near the annulus does not exist, the excision can be made on a hypothetical ribbon relatively close to the annulus. This is to prevent inadvertent excision of a portion of the annulus as such severe calcification may cause damage to the annulus and part of it may be inadvertently removed. A polymer aortic valve prosthesis is designed and fabricated slightly smaller (normally 1–2 mm smaller) in diameter than the diameter of the patient's annulus. The sinuses are removed in a way that only a rim of aortic

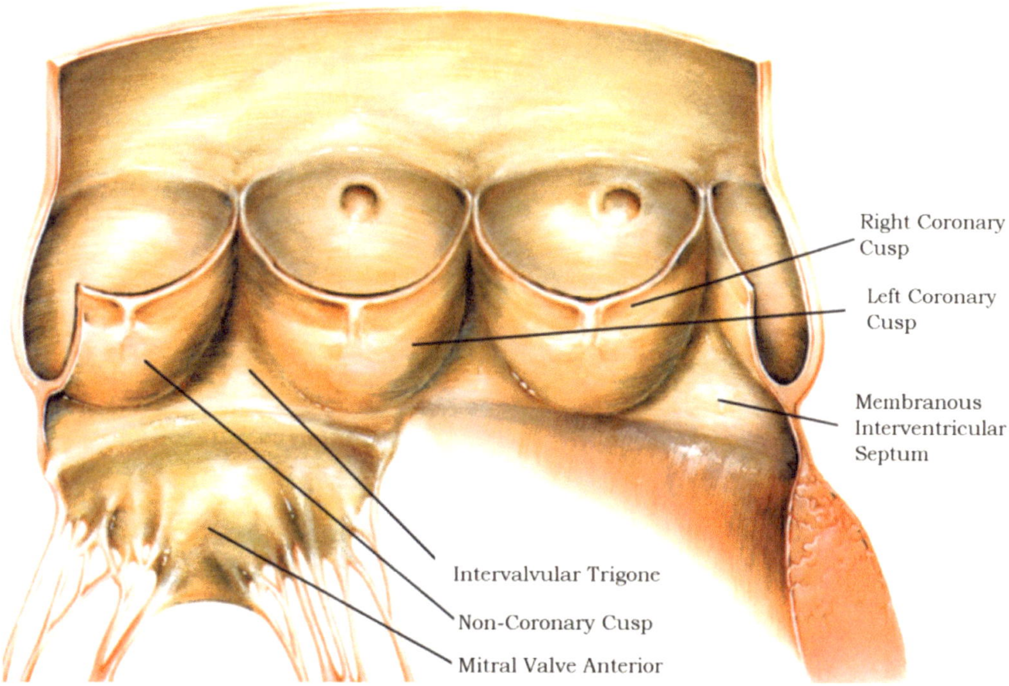

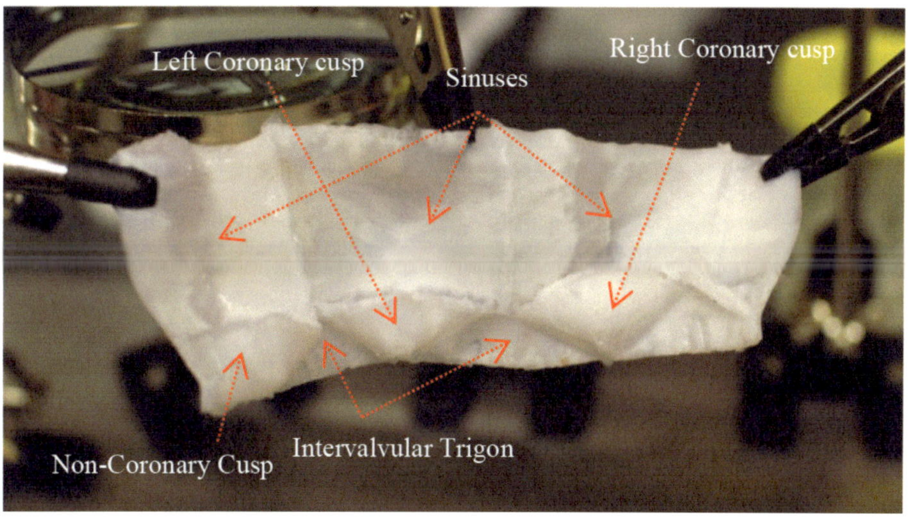

Figure 7. Demonstration of an opened out view of the aortic valve to illustrate the subvalvular anatomy. As the left ventricle has a common inlet and outlet, the anatomy of the aortic valve and mitral valve is intimately related. The top image is a typical diagram of the opened out ascending aorta including the aortic valve and the lower image is the synthetic ascending aorta proposed in this study which is one piece of the aortic root including the valve and coronary outlets.

wall above the cusps remains. Three sutures are placed through the prosthesis and the patient's annulus (**Figure 8A1**, **2** and **B1**, **2**) and the prosthesis is then lowered into the patient's annulus and inverted into the left ventricle (**Figure 8B3**). The sutures should then be run

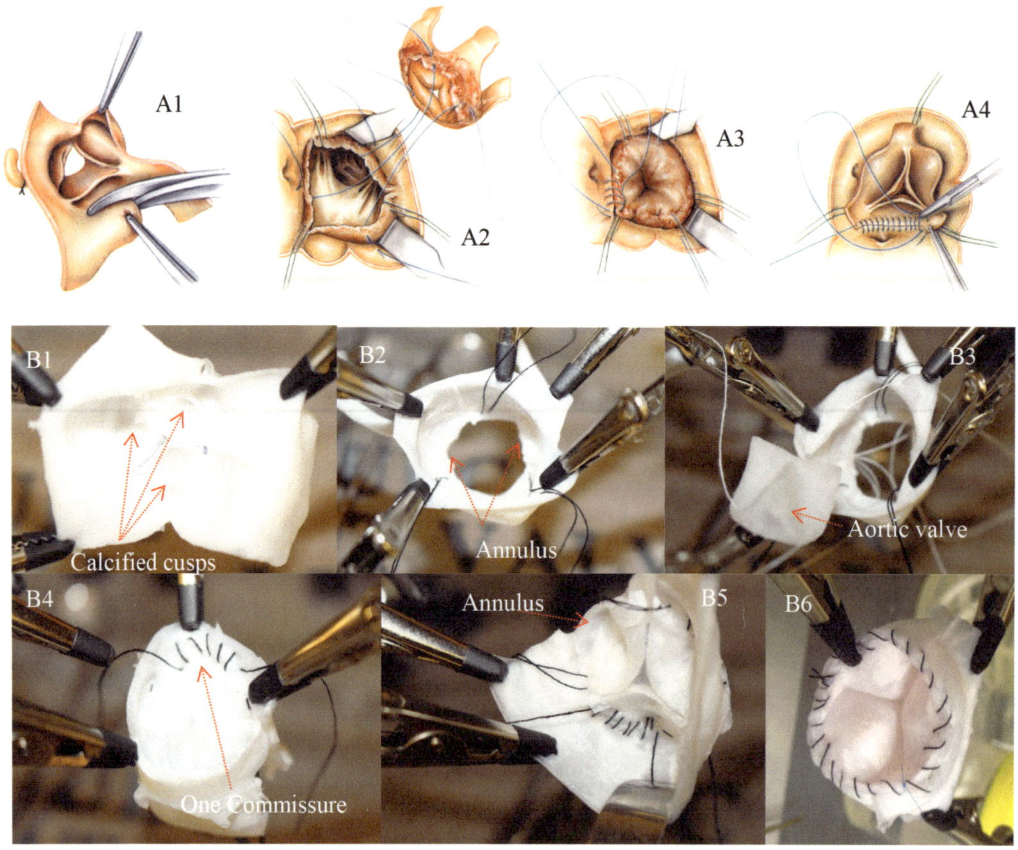

Figure 8. Anastomosis procedure of the prosthetic aortic valve and the ascending aorta built in this study. (1) The sinuses are removed in a way that only a rim of aortic wall above the cusps is left as shown in A1 and B1, (2) the calcific leaflets are removed as described above (B2), (3) three sutures are placed through the prosthesis and the patient annulus for guiding the valve into the right position in annulus, (4) the valve is anchored to the annulus. As shown almost one commissure is attached (A3, A4 and B4, showing the attachment from the aortic side, B5, showing the attachment from the ventricular side) and sutures are carried around to complete the anastomosis (B6).

toward each commissure and firmly tied ensuring the suture line is kept slightly below the patient's annulus. In the case of bioprosthesis, special care must be taken to avoid the conduction tissue under the commissure between the right coronary and the noncoronary cusps, however this is not required for the polymeric valve. Following this, the valve is then everted and sutures are initiated at the low points of the sinuses and are brought up to the commissures (**Figure 8A3**, **4** and **B4–B6**) [9].

2.1.6. Congenital aortic stenosis

The left and right cusps are fused together at the commissure which is considered as a relative underdevelopment of the right coronary leaflet (cusp) and the orifice is typically a cut between the left- and noncoronary cusps. The commissure between these two cusps is typically well-developed, however the other commissure may be dissimilar in degree of development and may merely be a primitive raphe. A simple incision is typically made in one (or two) commissure(s) of the right coronary leaflets (cusps). Incision of the other commissure may depend on its degree of development as well as the extension and depth of the right coronary leaflet (cusp).

2.1.7. *Surgical procedure*

In the first step, a transverse aortotomy is prepared and the valve is uncovered with small cusp retractors. Forceps are used to hold the leaflets and an incision is made on the well-developed commissure all the way to the annulus (**Figure 9A1** and **A2**). The assessment is carefully made on the depth of support and the degree of development of the right coronary leaflet. Due to the fact that the right coronary leaflet develops a coaptation area with the other leaflets (and not prolapse), the other commissure is carefully incised. In the last step, the subvalvular area is carefully checked to ensure there is no subvalvular stenosis underneath. The procedure on the proposed synthetic model is shown in **Figure 9B1–B4**.

2.2. Part B: coronary artery bypass surgery

The wall thicknesses of the coronary arteries possess a range from 0.42 to 1.35 mm [10]. The thickness of the saphenous vein wall is approximately 0.79 ± 20 μm [11] and the outer diameter of the lower bound coronary artery is 1.2 mm [12], whereas the diameter of the upper bound harvested saphenous vein is 7 mm with a normal minimum diameter of 3.6 mm and a normal maximum diameter of 4.84 mm within one vessel length [12].

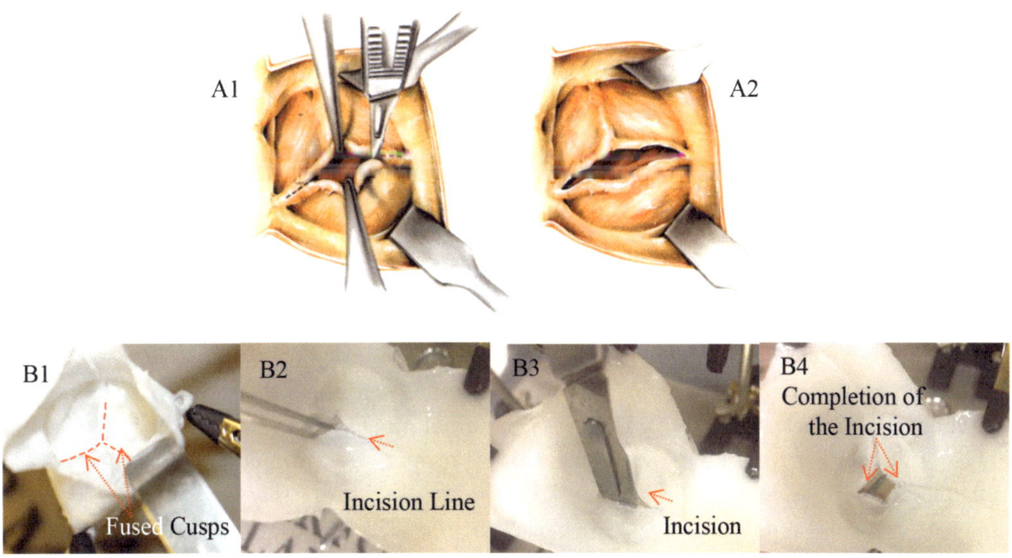

Figure 9. The exposure of the valve and incision of the well-developed commissure all the way back to the annulus (A1, A2)—top view. In the synthetic model, initially all three cusps are fused together. The practice is to make the main incision as discussed in the manuscript. (1) The valve is exposed (B1), (2) the incision line is determined (B2), (3) the incision is made all the way back to the annulus (B3) and (4) the incision is completed (B4).

2.2.1. Cryogel preparation

Polyvinyl alcohol cryogel (PVA-c), 99+% (Sigma-Aldrich) hydrolyzed with a molecular weight of 146,000–186,000 was implemented for the solution preparation which is outlined in more detail in our previous studies [10, 11]. The proposed cryogel material requires a thermal cycling procedure in order to physically crosslink the long molecules. Therefore, the design is limited to molds that can be implemented with the anti-freeze cooling bath which takes place within ethylene glycol solution with a temperature change of −20 to +20°C [12].

2.2.2. Mold design

Ten sizes of arteries, ranging from 1.5 to 7 mm are targeted in order to provide for all of the possible sizes implemented in CABG, which also includes internal mammary artery (IMA), saphenous vein (SVG) and radial artery (RA) grafting. The normal internal diameter for the human saphenous vein is 1.75 mm (without distention) and 2.18 mm (with distension) [5]. The diameter of artery and vein cores chosen for the design are from 1 to 2.5 mm. The length the vessels is simplified to a 10 cm long graft of continuous diameter and a wall thickness with no alterations.

In order to attain the precise dimensions, a flat plate design was implemented. This design consists of two flat symmetrical plates with the dimensions of each artery size fixed into a semicircular channel. When these compartments mate, a cylindrical graft is made (**Figure 10a** and **b**).

Another main issue addressed by this design is the capability for the cores to always remain concentric with the mold cavity. Our exclusive solution is to implement tension in the cores through a conical centering system. This feature ensures the cores remain centered regardless of orientation or disturbance imparted on the mold during the fabrication process. The conical mechanism is designed with a 45° taper on each end of the cylinder (**Figure 10c**).

2.2.3. Mold fabrication

The 3D rendering of the mold was fabricated on SolidWorks R2016 software. Renderings were printed using a Mojo (Proto 3000, Mississauga, Canada) 3D printer with a resolution between layers of 100 μm.

2.2.4. PVA cryogel models

The proposed material has similar mechanical properties to those of the coronary artery tissue. The molds were packed with 10% PVA-c and the final models were fabricated. These models are close in geometry and have similar mechanical properties to that of native tissues and are suitable to model vasculature for the simulation of bypass surgery (**Figure 11**). The circumferential strength of the proposed models reported here is 0.50 ± 0.12 MPa which is comparable to the native tissue (0.39 ± 0.07 MPa) [13, 14] with less than 5% discrepancy.

Using this procedure, vessels with a mean outer diameter of 1.30 mm and a mean luminal diameter of 600 μm can be produced where the dimension of the vessel thickness is 350 μm. These vessels have a normal vessel length of 60 mm and thus, vessels have efficaciously been

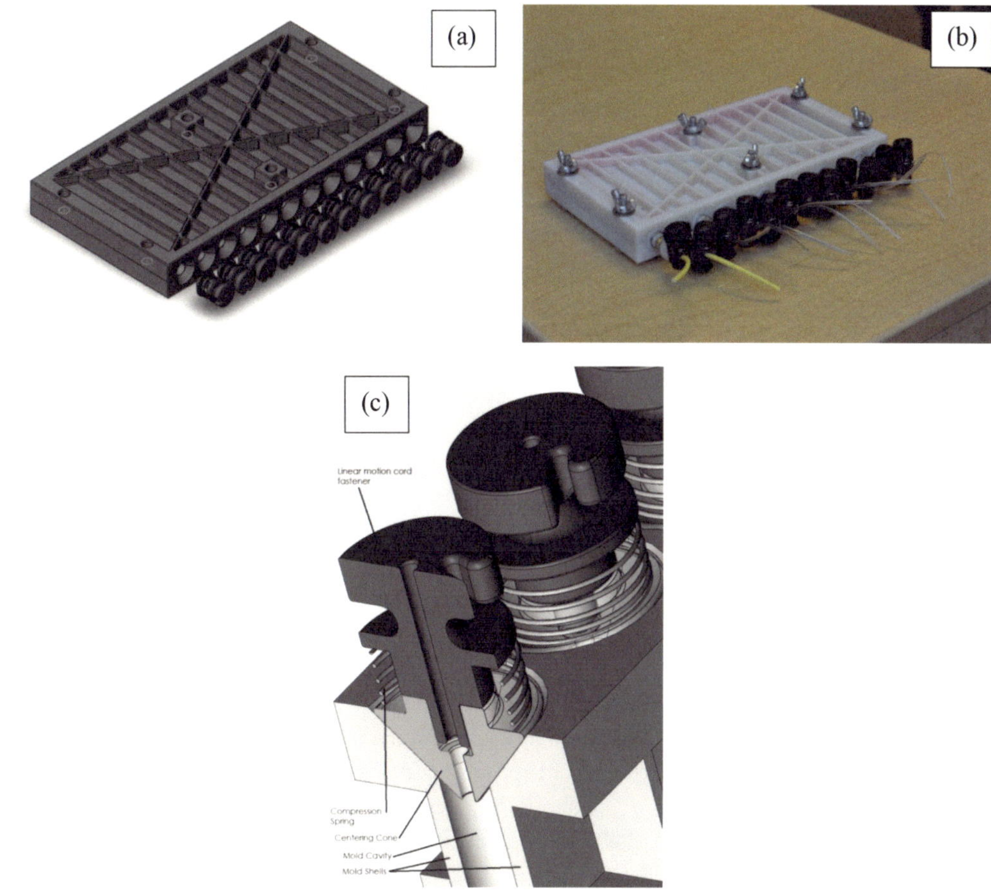

Figure 10. (a) CAD design, (b) the prototype of the mold for the construction of synthetic grafts. Twelve grafts with variations of sizes are developed in the same batch and (c) tensioning mechanism, the conic fixture holds the cord constantly at the center and the spring behind it is for providing a minimal tension on the cord so it is continuously under stretch [17].

fabricated in small scales. We have the capability of reliably creating vessels with a diameter ranging from 1.5 to 7 mm, **Figure 11** and **Table 1**.

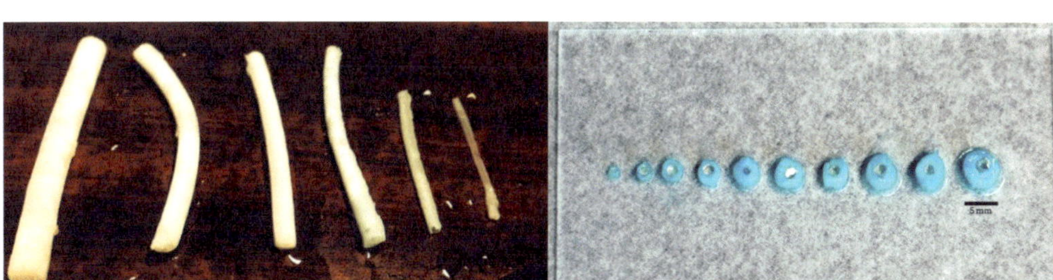

Figure 11. The models of synthetic manufactured grafts made of 10% PVA-c [17].

OD (outer diameter) (mm)	Thickness
1.5	350 μm
2.1	500 μm
2.9	670 μm
3.4	820 μm
4.2	940 μm
4.8	1.2 mm
5.5	1.4 mm
6.1	1.8 mm
7	2.0 mm

Table 1. Sizes of the proposed synthetic [17].

2.2.5. End to side anastomosis

We utilized a range of prolene (polypropylene) sutures (size: 2.0–6.0). The dull-witted marginal is incised with scissors (**Figure 12a**). A suture is passed (1) through the arterial wall, (2) through the vein and (3) through the arterial wall and (4) tagged. The other end is (1) brought through the vein and (2) the vein is again lowered into place. (3) The suture line is brought up to the right side. (4) The other suture is brought through the heel of the vein, (5) through the artery, (6) up the left side and around the toe, thus, completing the suture line, **Figure 12b**. In the end (7) a cannulation is utilized to ensure an excellent connection of the graft to the artery (**Figure 12c–e**).

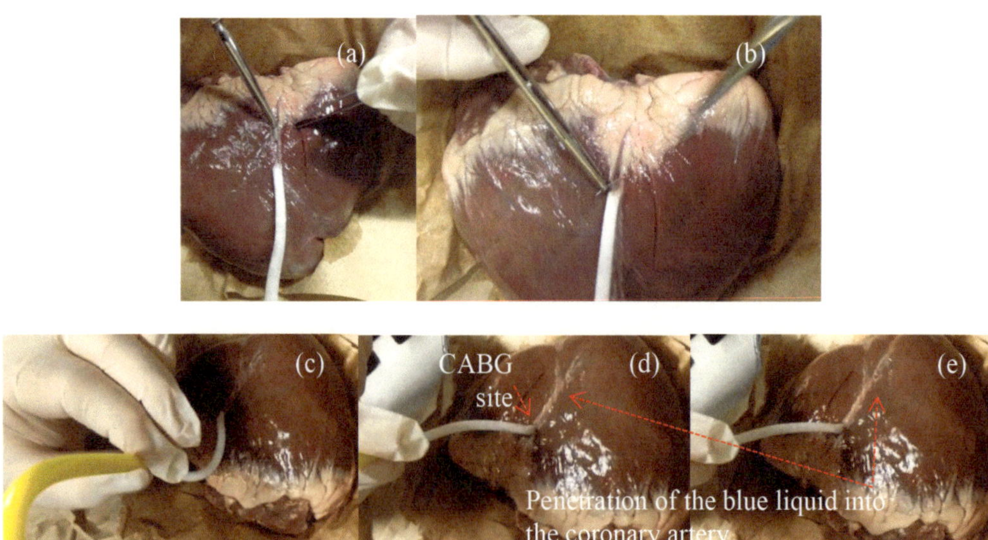

Figure 12. Anastomosis of a graft to coronary artery on a pig heart. (a) Groundwork on the coronary artery and the approximation of the location of anastomosis, (b) the suturing graft to the location of anastomosis, (c), (d) and (e) represent the cannulation test. Blue water is perfused through graft by applying a suitable pressure and the location of anastomosis is tested and observed for leaks [17].

2.2.6. Side-to-side anastomosis

We utilized a range of prolene (polypropylene) suture of the same size. The grafts are organized, **Figure 13a**. Both grafts A and B are notched longitudinally, **Figure 13b**. The incision must be accurate as an unsuitable incision may cause narrowing on the graft at the location of anastomosis. The suturing procedure follows the same routine (**Figure 13c–f**). (1) A suture is guided inside-outside the artery on graft A and (2) labeled. (3) The suture line is brought up inside-outside the vein on graft B and (4) outside-inside the artery on graft A (**Figure 13g** and **h**). (5) The suture is brought up outside-inside the vein on graft B and (6) inside-outside the artery on graft A and (7) around the end of arteriotomy to complete the anastomosis (**Figure 13i**) [15, 16].

There are other methods which can be implemented for the side-to-side or the end-to-end anastomosis as shown in **Figure 14a** and **b** are not explained in detail.

In the final step, side-to-side anastomosis of a small-scale graft to the ascending aorta was simulated, **Figure 15**. The ascending aorta implemented in this study is made of the cryogel biomaterials,

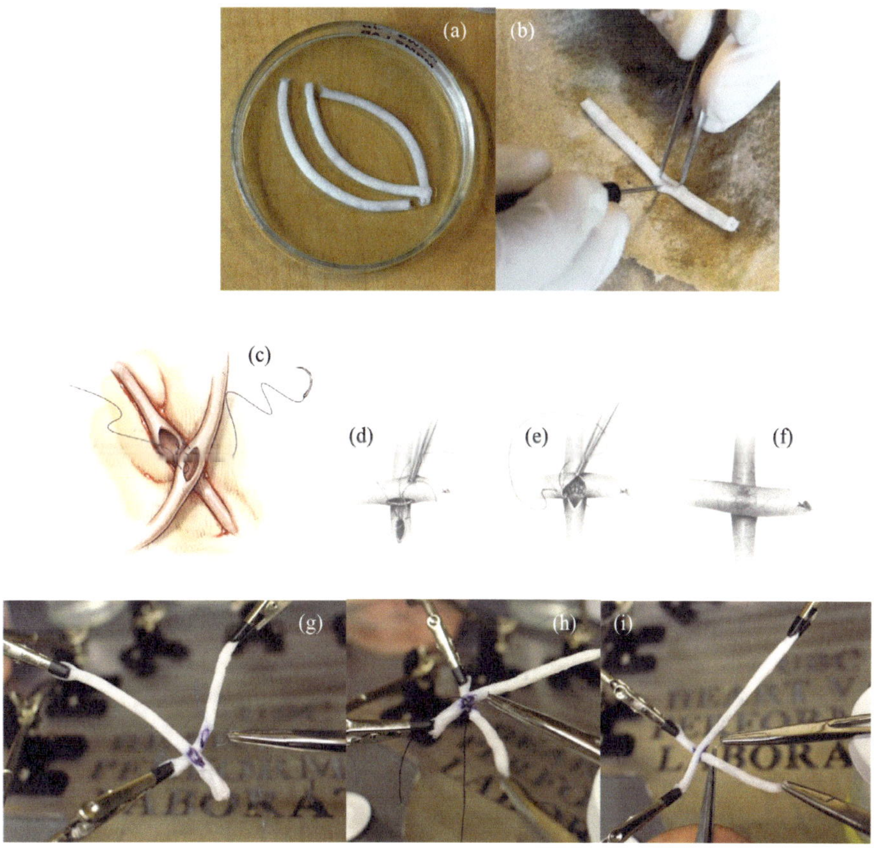

Figure 13. Presentation of side–to-side anastomosis. (a) Three synthetic grafts implemented in this study. (b) Presentation of applying a longitudinal incision, (c) presentation of a side-to-side anastomosis ideally, (d)–(f) are the recommended stages for the side-to-side anastomosis [12], (g) corresponding to stage (d) on the graft, (h) corresponding to stage (e) on the graft and (i) achievement of the anastomosis on the graft [17].

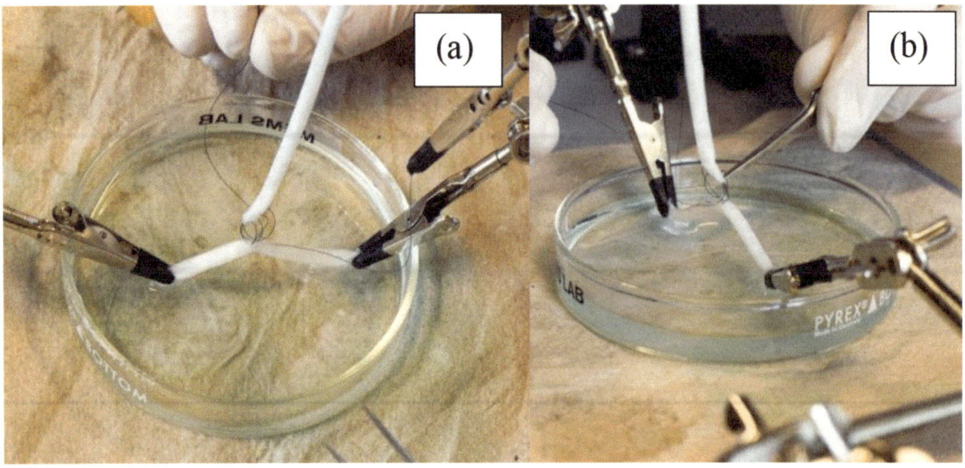

Figure 14. (a) Other methods implemented for the side-to-end anastomosis and (b) end-to-end anastomosis, both on the synthetic platforms [17].

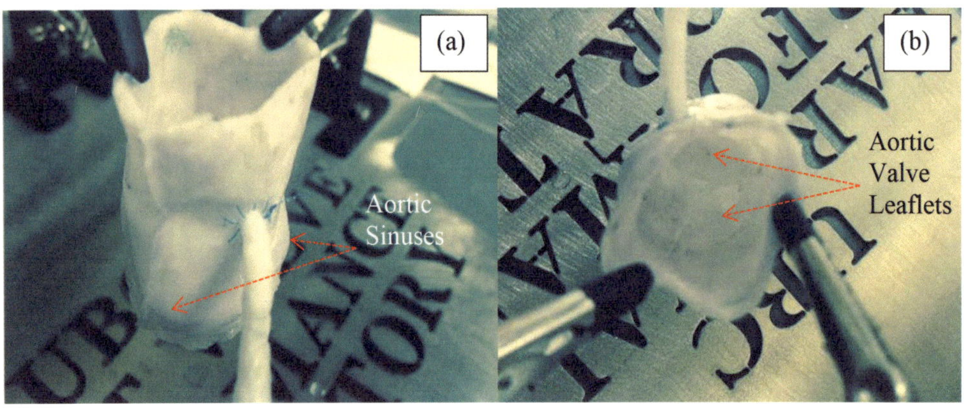

Figure 15. (a) Simulation of the side-to-side anastomosis of a small-scale graft to the valve conduit and (b) top view of the valve conduit and the small graft.

however possessed mechanical properties close to those of the leaflet tissue and the valve conduit. This model contains the sinuses and the aortic valve placed in a singular piece. Then, side-to-side anastomosis of a small graft to the valve conduit was attained using the proposed platform.

3. Conclusion

This chapter summarizes a novel emerging technology by which a complex surgery can be accurately simulated. We proposed a novel model of the ascending aorta made of synthetic material which maintains similar mechanical properties and geometry to that of native tissue by which a complicated heart valve replacement surgery can be simulated step-by-step.

It is known that available surgical simulators lack fidelity or are not adequately lifelike, though in this chapter a high fidelity platform was designed and fabricated. This platform may be used by young surgical residents or cardiac surgeons to develop expertise on the matter. More platforms will be developed so that other valve and ascending aorta related surgeries such as Yacob, David or Bentall procedures can be precisely simulated in a similar fashion.

Additionally to the best of the authors' knowledge, for the first time a platform for fabricating artificial cryogel micro-vessels is demonstrated in order to address a lack of availability to coronary artery bypass practice materials. Previously, small cryogel vessels did not exist simply because of their complicated geometries. The vessels presented feature a biomaterial with mechanical properties and geometries which are not statistically different from human vessels and the models have been productively implemented to model a coronary artery bypass surgical procedure. The penetration ability and resistance to rupture the sutures with the diverse range of sizes from 2.0 to 6.0 was verified and deemed acceptable using prolene (polypropylene) suture. The proposed material appears to be well-matched with polyglactin (vicryl) sutures as well [17].

For forthcoming work, the suture penetrating ability and resistance to rupture by associating diverse sutures polyglactin (vicryl) versus prolene 5-0/6-0/7-0) by means of a semi-quantitative scoring method will be modeled. Suture retention by utilizing pull test data compared to the real tissues can be also considered. A short case study showing the appropriateness of the cryogel vessels in a virtual model to educate operators and its outcomes (which is essentially semi-quantitative scoring methods) will be implemented. The accessibility of practice tools for surgeons will contribute to improve their adroitness and self-reliance in cardiothoracic surgery.

Acknowledgements

The authors acknowledge the University of British Columbia and NSERC (Discovery Grant) for financial support.

Author details

Emily Earl and Hadi Mohammadi*

*Address all correspondence to: hadi.mohammadi@ubc.ca

The Heart Valve Performance Laboratory, School of Engineering, Faculty of Applied Science, University of British Columbia, Kelowna, BC, Canada

References

[1] Paulis D, Scaffa R, Forlani S, Chiariello L. The Valsalva graft in aortic valve repair and replacement. Cardiothoracic Surgery. 2005;**2005**(1129):1-9

[2] Millon LE, Mohammadi H, Wan WK. Anisotropic polyvinyl alcohol (PVA) for cardiovascular applications. Journal of biomedical materials research (B). 2006;**79B**(2):305-311

[3] Wan WK, Millon LE, Mohammadi H. Anisotropic Cryogels for Cardiovascular Application. US Patent 9,096,744 B2 (2015)

[4] Mohammadi H, Mequanint K. Prosthetic aortic heart valves: Modeling and design. Medical Engineering & Physics. 2011;**33**(2):131-147

[5] Mohammadi H, Bahramian F, Wan W. Advanced modeling strategy for the analysis of heart valve leaflet tissue mechanics using high-order finite element method. Medical Engineering & Physics. 2009;**31**(9):1110-1117

[6] Mohammadi H. Nanocomposite biomaterial mimicking aortic heart valve leaflet mechanics. Proceedings of the Institution of Mechanical Engineers. Part H, Journal of Engineering in Medicine. 2011;**225**(7):718-722

[7] Mohammadi H, Boughner D, Millon LE, Wan WK. Design and simulation of a poly(vinyl alcohol)—Bacterial cellulose nanocomposite mechanical aortic heart valve prosthesis. Proceedings of the Institution of Mechanical Engineers. Part H, Journal of Engineering in Medicine. 2009;**223**(6):697-711

[8] Mohammadi H. Design and simulation of mechanical heart valve prostheses. ProQuest Diss Theses: University of Western Ontario; 2009

[9] Little AG, Merrill WH. Complications in Cardiothoracic Surgery: Avoidance and Treatment. The United States: John Wiley & Sons; 2009

[10] Zhao J, Jesper J, Yang J, Steen Rasmussen B, Liao D, Gregersen H. Manual pressure distension of the human saphenous vein changes its biomechanical properties-implication for coronary artery bypass grafting. Journal of Biomechanics. 2007;**40**:2268-2276

[11] Leask RL, Butany J, Johnston KW, Ethier CR, Ojha M. Human saphenous vein coronary artery bypass graft morphology, geometry and hemodynamics. Annals of Biomedical Engineering. 2005;**33**(3):301-309

[12] Wan WK, Millon LE, Mohammadi H. Anisotropic hydrogels for use in tissue replacement and reconstruction, bioagent entrapment and delivery, therapy pads and other medical goods. U.S. and International PCT Provisional Patents (2005), (US No.2005/60/666,316-PCT No.2006/000477)

[13] Millon LE, Mohammadi H, Wan WK. Anisotropic polyvinyl alcohol hydrogel for cardiovascular applications. Journal of Biomedical Materials Research-Part B Applied Biomaterials. 2006;**79**(2):305-311

[14] Kieser TM, Lewin AM, Graham MM, et al. Outcomes associated with bilateral internal thoracic artery grafting: The importance of age. The Annals of Thoracic Surgery. 2011;**92**:1269-1275 discussion 1275-6

[15] Elmistekawy EM, Gawad N, Bourke M, et al. Is bilateral internal thoracic artery use safe in the elderly? Journal of Cardiac Surgery. 2012;**27**:1-5

[16] Mohammadi H, Nestor B, Fradet G. Simulation of anastomosis in coronary artery bypass surgery. Journal of Cardiovascular Engineering and Technology. 2016;**7**(4):432-438

Chapter 7

Learning and Teaching after 50 Years of THORAX Surgery

Jaime Villalba Caloca, Avelina Sotres Vega,
Javier Pineda Gutiérrez, Sergio Martínez Fonseca,
Marcelino Alonso Gómez and
Bettina Sommer Cervantes

Additional information is available at the end of the chapter

http://dx.doi.org/10.5772/intechopen.72915

Abstract

Surgeries are practiced in different areas, and specifically in the thorax described in this chapter, the medical doctors must know in detail the biological structures in which they perform such surgical procedures. Therefore, in this chapter, we refer to the descriptive and topographical anatomy written by French doctors L. Testut and A. Latarjet. In earlier times, for several reasons, the medical surgeon operated all body organs and was involved in resolving the pathology of different areas. Currently and in the future, medical knowledge in thoracic surgery will cover subspecialties specifically divided, for example: assisted video surgery, interventional bronchoscopy, and mediastinoscopies to take mediastinal biopsies using robotic surgery of pulmonary exeresis to shorten the hospitalization period and even the days spent in the intensive care unit.

Keywords: surgery, thorax, education

1. Introduction

In the past, the assessment of surgical education started with the difficult acquisition of knowledge, reading through a total of six anatomy volumes published by Testut and Jacob and Testut and Latarjet. Besides, an unlimited number and type of general surgical procedures had to be carried out. Currently, surgical practice is mainly obtained through experimental models. These methods of teaching and learning surgical skills have shown that "if students outlive" the anatomical and functional steps, they will gain a greater understanding of anatomy and physiology. Nonetheless, surgeons must get a specific surgical specialty. In the future, surgeons will become subspecialists with genetic and robotic multitraining. However, it must be said that this issue may contain sensible medical ethical dilemmas, although this discipline derived from philosophy has grown in a very important way and surely will continue growing every day, mainly because of the positive impact of technological development on human well-being.

Regarding surgery, in the past, surgeons without any surgical specialty were capable of performing incisions in all cavities; they could correctly perform surgeries in the central nervous system, resolve cardiopathies, and dissect the abdomen. Currently, for instance in chest surgery, there are many subspecialties such as video-assisted surgery or interventional bronchoscopy performing surgeries such as pleural decortication, pulmonary resection, oncologic surgery, endocavitary aspiration, and transbronchial punctures for therapeutic, diagnostic or palliative purposes, and lately long-distance surgery and robotic surgery. The large number of subspecialties that have currently been added to pneumology, such as thoracic oncology, pulmonary pathophysiology, and intensive care of sleeping disorders, is worth noting. In addition to technological changes, in the future, thoracic surgeons will have to have knowledge/comprehend and support genomic medicine, molecular biology, epigenetics, computer networks, telecommunications, bioelectronics, artificial intelligence, communication and psychomedical techniques of treatment, geriatrics, preventive medicine, administration and health economics as well as ethics. Currently, thoracic surgery in the future will be practiced by groups of subspecialists that will need to be competent to select/have to choose from millions of data published daily in order to obtain and classify information.

2. From pulmonary collapse to video-assisted and robotic surgery

"Writing about general chest surgery practiced since 50 years ago to date, and its future trends is to describe the medical-surgical fight against two important diseases: in the past, against pulmonary tuberculosis, and currently, against lung cancer. In the future, the challenge will be to unify video-assisted approach and robotics along with research and study of new drugs against these two diseases" [1].

Pulmonary tuberculosis or "the great white plague" was a serious public health problem worldwide since time immemorial, as confirmed by the forensic analysis of human remains showing signs of tuberculosis.

If we remember and think about Thomas Mann's classic book "The Magic Mountain," which began to be written in 1912 and was finished in 1924 and which describes the hospitals that existed in the mountains of Switzerland, we may recognize that in those times it was suggested that the air that could be breathed at those heights was a good treatment for the white plague. The hospital most talked about is the Walls Sanatorium in Davos, where lung collapse measures were used to treat tuberculosis patients. Nowadays, some of those homes once inhabited by patients with Koch bacillus, became fashion great luxury hotels.

The National Institute of Respiratory Diseases in Mexico (NIRDM) was inaugurated in 1936 as the Huipulco Tuberculosis Sanatorium (**Figure 1**), a place where most patients suffered

http://dx.doi.org/10.5772/intechopen.72915

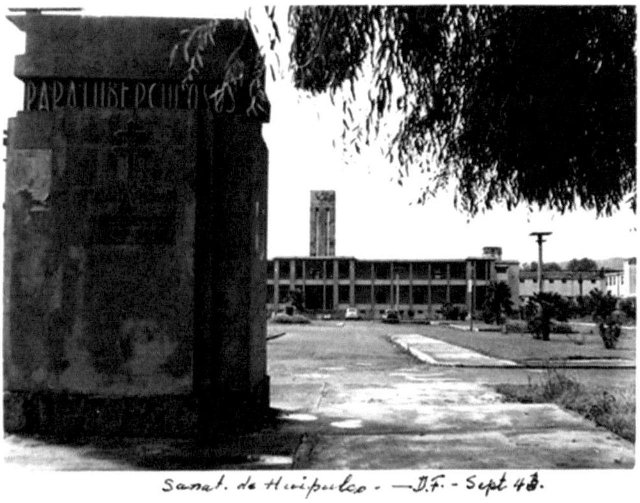

Figure 1. Huipulco tuberculosis sanatorium, Mexico City, 1936.

from pulmonary tuberculosis. The sanatorium was architecturally designed in such a way that the rooms for patients had only three and a half walls to allow the free cycling of fresh air. NIRDM was built approximately 15 km away from the urban area, on green fields full of trees with temperatures ranging between 5 and 11°C [2].

Over the years, overpopulation and the consequent urban growth have caused environmental changes along with different ways of thinking about the treatment of some diseases, including tuberculosis. Because tuberculosis has been earmarked with lower income, less financial resources are allotted to its treatment while much more money is allocated to chronic-degenerative diseases.

In the past, young students′ restlessness and an unreal desire to dress in the surgeon's uniform made the work even harder. The process was relatively slow since during the period as a medical student and specifically during the first 2 years, two tremendous subjects had to be studied exhaustively: the first one was descriptive anatomy. This task implied using "The Treatise on Descriptive Human Anatomy" by Testud and Jacob as a bedside book. The second subject was topographic anatomy based on "The Compendium of Topographic Anatomy" by Testut and Latarjet, a textbook that described human anatomy by regions.

Currently, much functional knowledge of the human body is mainly obtained in a practical way, either through experimental models or with dummies that had shown that "if students outlive" the anatomical and functional study steps, they will indisputably gain a greater understanding of anatomy and physiology knowledge.

When a medical student studies, learns clinical subjects such as pneumology, gastroenterology, or cardiology among other subjects, he or she does it closely to his or her tutor. The semiological study of the patient is performed on the analysis of the patient's symptoms, that is, if the patient presents clinical signs such as dyspnea or cough, lung anatomy will be remembered, as well as the physiology of the lower airways regarding ventilation, perfusion, and diffusion; the surgical coil will especially be thought about when procuring the patient's benefit. I think that in the future, all surgical/medical decisions will have to be taken by a group of experts, and a biologist-immunologist must be considered as one of them.

As for surgery, in the past, it was said that "the great surgeons made large incisions." Furthermore, these great surgeons surgically intervened all the organs of the different cavities of the human body, and, as I experienced while I was a medical student, I saw the same surgeon from The General Hospital of Mexico practicing surgeries very dexterously in the central nervous system, or to alleviate heart diseases as well as the most frequent procedures practiced in the abdomen, such as colicystectomies and intestinal resections.

When I was in the fourth year of my Bachelor's studies in medicine, I started studying the respiratory apparatus. It was the time when several types of thoracoplasty and some pulmonary resections were performed. After entering the surgery and seeing the surgical technique of thoracoplasty and the type of anesthesia used, I was impressed by the incision at the skin level, by the muscular separation, the entrance to the pleural cavity, and the desperiostization of the first, second and third ribs. So I decided to learn the surgical method and the postoperative management of this irreversible pulmonary collapse. Likewise, observing pulmonary resection was surprising too, due to the dissection of the pulmonary hilum and by the different techniques used to close the lobular bronchus or the lung.

In Mexico, Koch's bacillus caused severe damage to the population, and around 1890s, health authorities and the distinguished physician Eduardo Liceaga started an organization to fight against the infection by *Mycobacterium tuberculosis*. Among their actions, they initiated a medical service called Observation and Treatment of Tuberculosis.

In 1905, The General Hospital of Mexico was inaugurated. There, two pavilions were assigned for tuberculosis patients only, and after the Mexican Revolution (1910), this pathology incidence increased because of the poverty increment after the armed conflict [1].

In those years, no specific treatment against *M. tuberculosis* was available and its therapeutic management was based on herbal medicine without any etiological basis, even though the causal agent of this millennial suffering had been discovered since 1882 by the German doctor Roberto Koch.

In those previous years, "pulmonary resections" were performed by placing the pulmonary hilum, either lobar or the whole lung, in a tourniquet, and a dissection was performed. True cunning was required in order to apply a tourniquet to the entire pulmonary hilum to perform the pneumonectomy. This surgery caused significant bleeding and bronchopleural fistulas with 25–30% of mortality rate. Indisputably, in order to practice a pneumonectomy, the surgeon must dissect the veins, artery, and bronchus either from the segment, the lobe, or the lung. Doctor Overholt, who intervened his patients in a face-down position on an operation table specially designed by him, insisted in the dissection of the pulmonary hilum. Leo Eloesser also supported this surgical procedure.

In 1882, the same year in which Robert Koch (**Figure 2**) discovered the causal agent of pulmonary tuberculosis, Carlo Forlanini devised intrapleural pneumothorax [3]. Since Koch's postulates have been valid for 135 years, it is worth remembering them:

1. The bacterial pathogen is isolated from sick animals and never from healthy animals.
2. Bacteria can be isolated, cultivated, and purified from sick animals.
3. If bacteria are inoculated into a healthy susceptible host, illness would occur.

In 1954, Dr. Miguel Jiménez Sánchez registered a book describing the doctrine of respiratory trauma very well. His intention was to prevent it and give rise to the collapse therapy. It is worth describing this concept in the words of Dr. Jiménez:

"By the action of the inspiratory muscles, the lung tissue is subjected to a centrifugal distension that increases during inspiration, but does not disappear in the expiratory phase, since, during this phase, it occupies a space much bigger than the corresponding to its true complete rest position, which is the total collapse of the viscera, in which its retraction force is annulled, a circumstance that does not occur "in vivo" due to the existence of the pleural attraction that keeps the lung in a state of constant distension in the vicinity of the costal wall. In other words, the lung during expiration (physiological rest) is in a state of centrifugal hyperdistention that increases during each inspiration by the mechanisms already indicated."

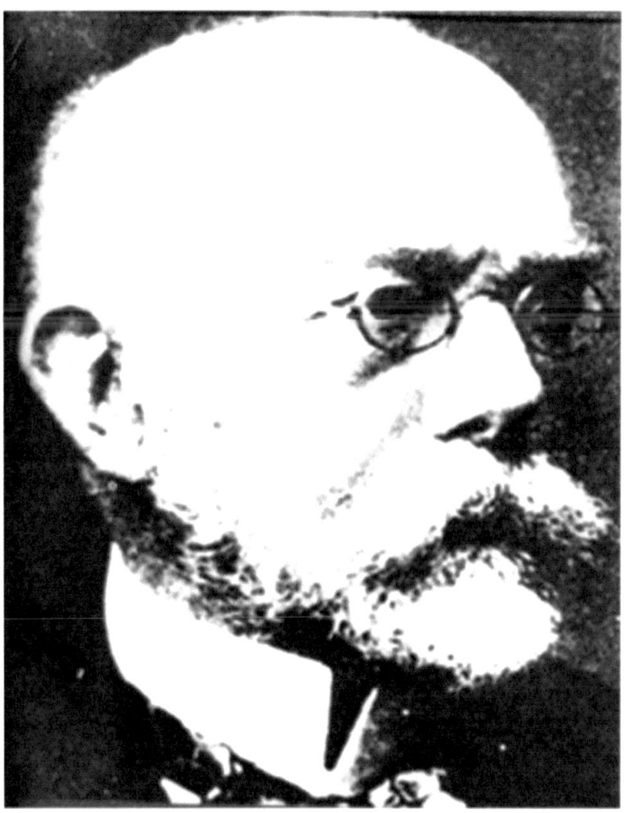

Figure 2. Robert Koch.

Also in the words of Dr. Jimenez: "The lung has a very delicate anatomical constitution and is formed of a tissue that is essentially elastic, uniform and eccentrically dilatable in the course of inspiration. It can be considered as a small elastic balloon that cannot dilate or retract as long as the inspiration does not allow the entrance of the air and the exhalation its exit. The alveolus is subjected to two opposing forces; on the one hand, the inspiratory muscles tend to dilate it, and on the other, the narrowing of the airways, by delaying the arrival of the air, oppose this dilatation. It is notable that a tissue as weak as that of the alveolus, due exclusively to its elastic expansion potential, can dampen the action of two opposing forces; and if its very delicate wall is not injured, it is that its dilatability is superior to the inspiratory dilation of the thorax" [4] (**Figure 3**).

These concepts described by Dr. Forlanini and established by Dr. Jimenez led to the idea that normal function became abnormal because of lung disease.

It must be mentioned that inflammatory factors generated by pulmonary infection develop pleuritis, since the pleural leaves are adhered, and because their function to impede lung collapse gets compromised, Dr. Forlanini implemented a surgical technique called "section of adhesions," to section them and avoid the lung's collapse. When this procedure was executed, the urethroscope was used because there was no other equipment (as, for instance, a pleuroscope) available to section the parieto-visceral adhesions.

With Dr. Forlanini's idea of causing pulmonary immobility, several physicians who treated pulmonary tuberculosis performed irreversible pulmonary collapse using different surgical techniques that comprised resection of the ribs in order to "letting the lung fall", that is, inducing pulmonary collapse and, consequently, improving mainly cavitary lesions.

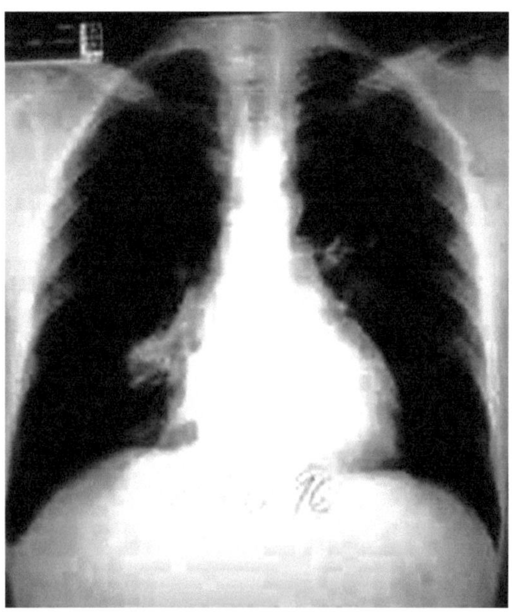

Figure 3. Right pneumothorax X-ray image.

Breathing is carried out through inspiration and expiration in a number of 12–18 breaths per minute in diseased lungs, and this gave Dr. Carlo Forlanini the notion of the respiratory trauma concept. He explained that in lungs infected with *M. tuberculosis,* the inspiration and expiration "beat" the lung parenchyma, therefore increasing the pulmonary injury, and his idea was to avoid the respiratory trauma through the intrapleural pneumothorax as far as possible.

The discovery of *M. tuberculosis* coincides with the concept that respiratory trauma caused the persistence of the pathology. Dr. Carlo Forlanini claimed that inspiration and exhalation hit the lung fundamentally on the thoracic area that he called "dominant lines" which he described in the diaphragm and in the pulmonary hilum areas, and he concluded that an injured lung suffered from respiratory trauma while the movement of inspiration and expiration did not affect the parenchyma of healthy lungs. Based on this idea, it was concluded that a measure for the treatment of pulmonary tuberculosis was to keep the patient at rest since it was a patient with respiratory trauma. To achieve this goal, different methods were conceived.

Subsequently, in Naples, Italy, Dr. Monaldi pursued the endocavitary aspiration to eliminate caseum from the tuberculous cavern, because the greatest amount of bacilli concentrates in that area [5].

Another surgical procedure practiced to avoid respiratory trauma was the phrenicectomy, although it caused respiratory insufficiency, paralysis of the hemidiaphragm, and therefore serious pulmonary ventilation problems.

In 1952, Waksman was awarded the Nobel Prize for his research in streptomycin discovery, a drug that fortunately led to a significant reduction in surgical measures for the treatment of pulmonary tuberculosis.

There are different procedure types of thoracoplasty as follows:

1. Total thoracoplasty.
2. Subtotal thoracoplasty.
3. Upper partial thoracoplasty.
4. Partial inferior thoracoplasty.
5. The widened thoracoplasty.
6. Iterative thoracoplasties.
7. Thoraco-apicolysis.

Frequently, pulmonary tuberculosis caused infection in the pleural cavity or empyema tuberculosis. In most cases, this pathological situation required draining of pleural pus through a water seal connected to suction. Furthermore, the pleura responded to the *M. tuberculosis* invasion with inflammation and thickening of both visceral and parietal leaves of the pleura; the lung remained "imprisoned" by the pleural response. Simultaneously, "pulmonary incarceration" caused ventilation disorders, and it was necessary to practice surgery and resect the "pleural shell," removing the tuberculosis pleura and improving ventilatory mechanics.

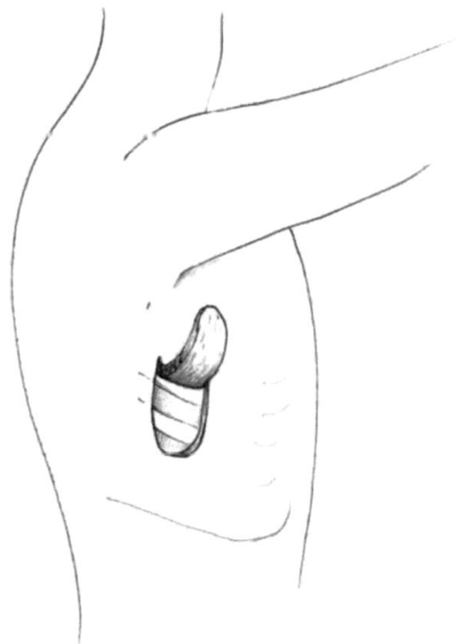

Figure 4. Eloesser's window technique for pleural drainage.

In 1935, Dr. Leo Eloesser devised a surgical technique called Eloesser's Window to drain the tuberculous empyema by opening the pleural cavity. This "window" was a $2 \times 3\ cm^2$ cut into the costal wall and thus allowing the cleaning of the cavity to perform the pulmonary decortication (**Figure 4**).

3. Plumbing, gel, and lucite balls

Extrapleural pneumolysis. To collapse the pulmonary apex, extrapleural pneumolysis was devised. It consists of lowering the "tip of the lung" via the extrapleural route to allow collapsing of the cavernous lesions of the upper pulmonary segments. One of the problems with this technique was to support the collapse of the vertex because the application of air was difficult due to the presence of fibrous tissue. This led to the inclusion of different materials as, for instance, lucite balls (similar to ping pong balls) into the extrapleural space to maintain the pulmonary collapse and facilitate the application of air into the extrapleural space.

Around 1933, Dr. Banyai, while trying to perform an intrapleural pneumothorax in a tuberculous patient, introduced air into the peritoneal cavity, causing a pneumoperitoneum (**Figure 5**) that enhanced the evolution of tuberculosis lesions in the inferior lung lobes. This gave rise to the fact that in certain topographic situations of the tuberculous lesions, the pneumoperitoneum will be used.

All surgical interventions, intrapleural pneumothorax, extrapleural pneumothorax (difficult to maintain), plumbing (**Figure 6**), lucite balls (**Figure 7**), phrenicectomy, pneumoperitoneum,

http://dx.doi.org/10.5772/intechopen.72915

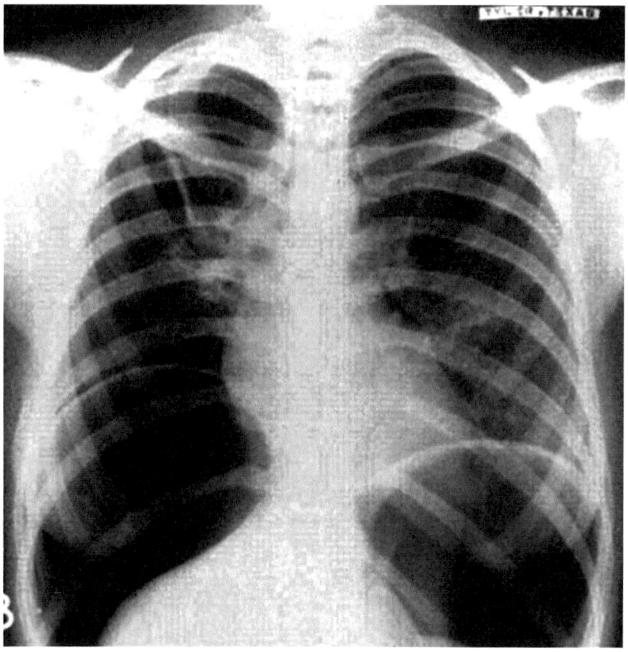

Figure 5. Pneumoperitoneum X-ray image.

and all types of thoracoplasty mentioned earlier are practiced to keep the lung at rest to avoid respiratory trauma.

Although nowadays, efficient primary and secondary drugs for tuberculosis treatment exist, the lack of education and low-economic income have contributed to bacillary resistance, and occasionally thoracic surgery must be practiced to maintain the lung at rest.

Undoubtedly, as it has been stated by well-known tisiology specialists "tuberculosis has been an excellent teacher and an important teaching and learning factor in the management and treatment of different diseases of the chest."

On the other hand, thoracoplasties consist of removing the posterior and lateral edges of the ribs, which are the parietal pleural support. This excision induced the lung collapse, and the surgical techniques are shown in **Table 1** [6].

Plumbing, a technique that consisted of the application of oil to provoke lung collapse and diminish the respiratory trauma, lowers the apex of the lung, and the introduction of lucite balls into the pleural cavity was also used to avoid respiratory trauma. These methods occasionally caused erosions of the bronchi; even though oil could be expulsed through air expulsion, the lucite balls had to be surgically removed.

Thoracoplasty was another surgical method used to reduce respiratory trauma. It consists of the resection of the first five ribs in two surgical times, from the vertebral joint to the sternum costal joint. All patients submitted to thoracoplasty had paradoxical breathing due to the lack

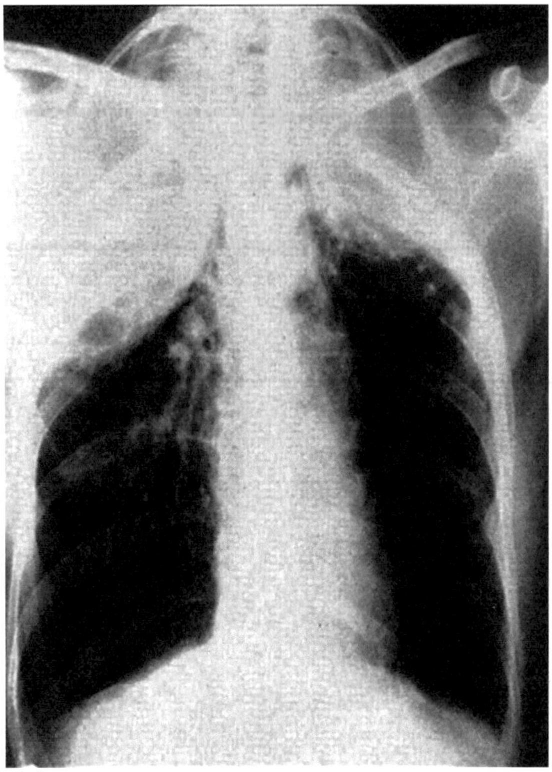

Figure 6. Plumbing X-ray image.

of support offered by the ribs, to the development of pleural adhesion, and to consequent negative pressure. These disturbances on the pulmonary ventilation "mediastinal swing and loss of costal support" invited the surgeon to practice a different type of thoracoplasty, that is, performing a partial resection of the ribs. This type of surgery, called chondroflexion, decreased the hemithorax space and no paradoxical breathing was produced (**Figure 8**).

In some patients, a post-thoracoplasty resection was prescribed in order to remove excavated lesions through lobar or segmental resection.

In addition to thoracoplasties, to keep the lung at rest, the phrenic nerve was sectioned with the purpose of paralyzing the corresponding hemidiaphragm and avoid trauma in the inferior dominant line. This surgery was performed for many years but unfortunately caused respiratory insufficiency because of diaphragmatic immobility and infections that were consequence of poor secretion management. In the long term, hemodynamic disorders such as pulmonary artery hypertension developed (**Figure 9**).

In Mexico City, the first lung resection was performed by Leo Eloesser at the Huipulco Tuberculosis Sanatorium (NIRD), and he was assisted by William B. Neff, who took care of the general anesthesia (**Figure 10**).

In the 1950s, staplers were developed in the Soviet Union to perform resections of pulmonary pathology in "wedge," that is, without dissecting the corresponding hilum. This surgical

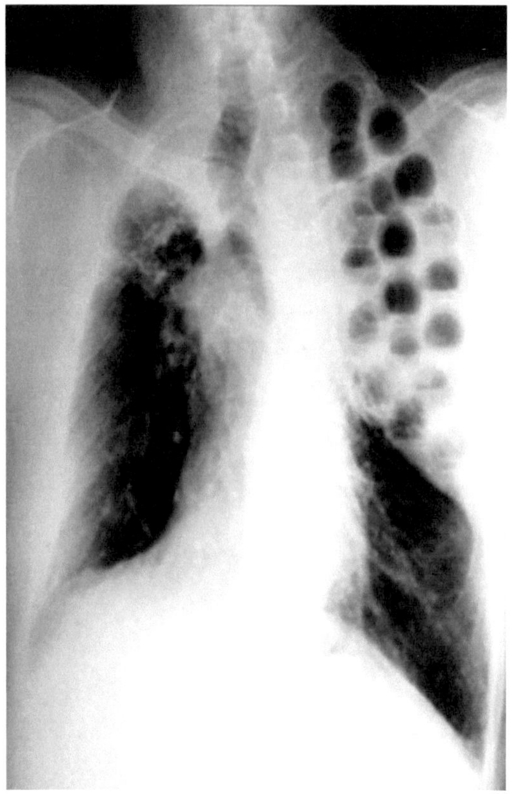

Figure 7. Lucite balls X-ray image.

method was used in the Soviet Union mainly due to the serious problem of pulmonary tuberculosis that they faced in addition to the lack of pleuropulmonary surgeons. Over time, these staplers were used less frequently to perform wedge resection but more often mainly to perform pulmonary resections stapling the bronchus only, to try to solve bronchial fistulas (**Figure 11**).

Pulmonary tuberculosis repeatedly causes pleural effusion due to infected pulmonary peripheral nodules. This situation causes tuberculous empyema and bronchopleural fistula. These patients with tuberculous empyema were handled by Dr. Leo Eloesser through a drainage of the pleural cavity to the outside, communicating the pleural cavity by means of a 2- or 3-cm opening to the outside. This technique facilitated the daily cleaning and healing of the pleural cavity, and due to the symphysis of the pleural leafs, there was no total pulmonary collapse. This surgical technique, called Eloesser, was generally followed by decortication of the pleural cavity and closure, if any, of the air leakage of the lung parenchyma. In the past, Eloesser's surgery in addition to antituberculosis drugs provided good results, and currently Eloesser's method continues to be performed from time to time (**Figures 12** and **13**).

The discovery of streptomycin by Waskman in 1943 was worth the Nobel Prize for Medicine and caused the surgical measures for the treatment of pulmonary tuberculosis to decrease significantly. Streptomycin sulfate is an aminoglycoside that has activity against aerobic gram-negative bacteria such as the tuberculosis bacillus. Streptomycin penetrates the cell

1. Intrapleural pneumothorax	
1882	Forlanini
1898	Murphy
1908	Saugman
1909	Brauer
1912	Jacobeus
2. Phrenic nerve palsy	
1911	Stüertz
1913	Sauerbruch
1920	Felix/Goetze
3. Thoracoplasty	
1907	Friedrich
1911	Wilms
1913	Sauerbruch
1922	Brauer
1925	Alexander
1935	Semb
1954	Björk
4. Extrapleural pneumolysis	
1891	Tuffer
1913	Baer
1936	Graff
5. Pneumoperitoneum	
1933	Banyai
	Klopstoc
	Vajda
1938	Bennet

Table 1. Surgery of pulmonary tuberculosis.

membrane of bacteria, fixes to the ribosome, and therefore does not stop the initiation of protein synthesis in bacteria. Unfortunately, in some cases, it causes renal failure and deafness, and patients receiving this antibiotic must be closely monitored.

3.1. Trachea

Tuberculosis patient's expectoration also affected the trachea producing ulcers and sometimes retraction by proliferation of connective tissue and stenosis. This, at least a 50-year-old

http://dx.doi.org/10.5772/intechopen.72915

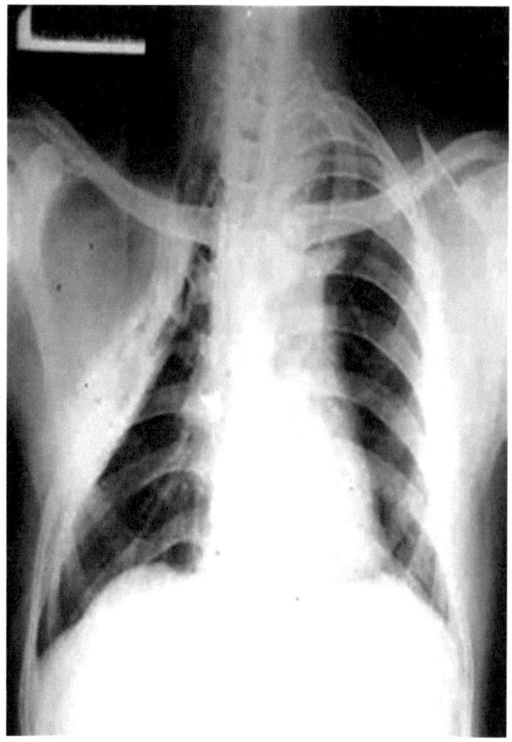

Figure 8. Right thoracoplasty X-ray image.

problem, was a very serious complication without antituberculosis drugs, since morbidity and mortality rates and low-economic income contributed to the failure of its surgical treatment. Dr. Hermes Grillo started tracheal surgery and devised different surgical techniques with good results. A very important contribution for the study of the trachea was made by Dr. Chevalier Jackson (1865–1958) who is considered the father of bronchoscopy and laryngoscopy; he designed rigid bronchoscopes and used them for diagnosis and bronchodilation (**Figure 14**).

Isoniazid was discovered in 1945; this drug inhibits the synthesis of mycolic acid on the wall of the bacteria. On the other hand, parasinosalicylic acid (PAS) is a bacteriostatic of the tuberculous bacillus, which is very useful in inhibiting or retarding bacterial resistance to streptomycin and isoniazid. With isoniazid, streptomycin, PAS, and ethambutol (1961), thoracic surgery decreased due to diminished indications in pulmonary tuberculosis therapies and new drug treatments.

It is impossible to explain and describe the surgical techniques of the past without mentioning some words about pulmonary tuberculosis. Pulmonary tuberculosis was the pathological condition that originated the art of its surgical management.

Currently, the prevalence of tuberculosis patients has decreased significantly, whereas diseases such as cancer, pulmonary fibrosis, and asthma have increased in a high percentage. In the future, chronic-degenerative diseases will dominate respiratory pathology, and so in

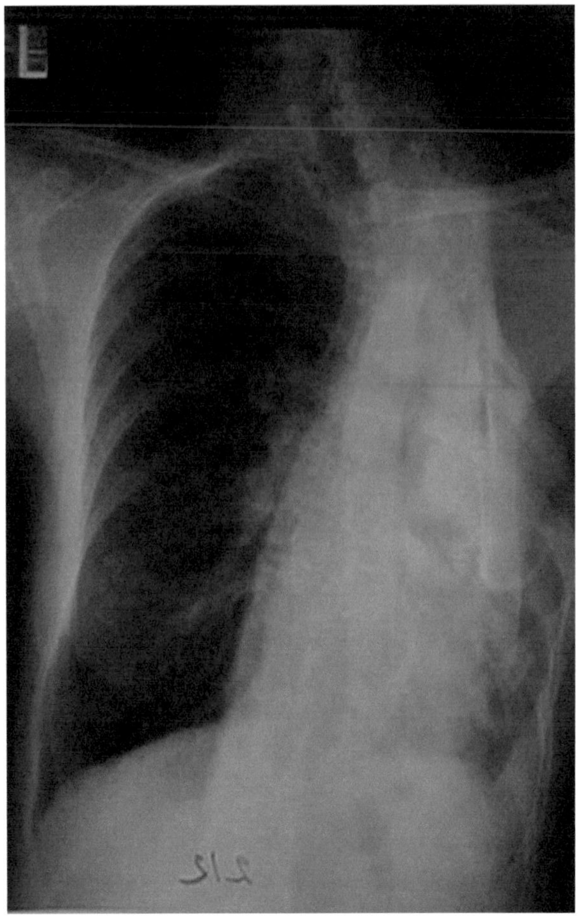

Figure 9. Left thoracoplasty X-ray image.

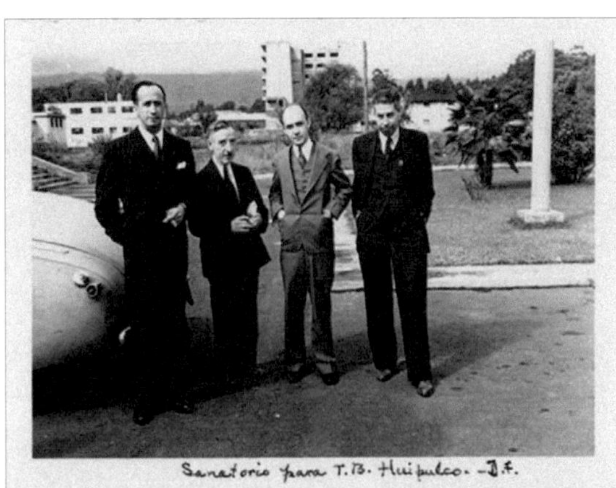

Figure 10. From right to left: Ismael Cosio Villegas, Leo Eloesser, William B. Neff, and Donato Alarcón at the National Institute of respiratory diseases (NIRD), Mexico City.

http://dx.doi.org/10.5772/intechopen.72915

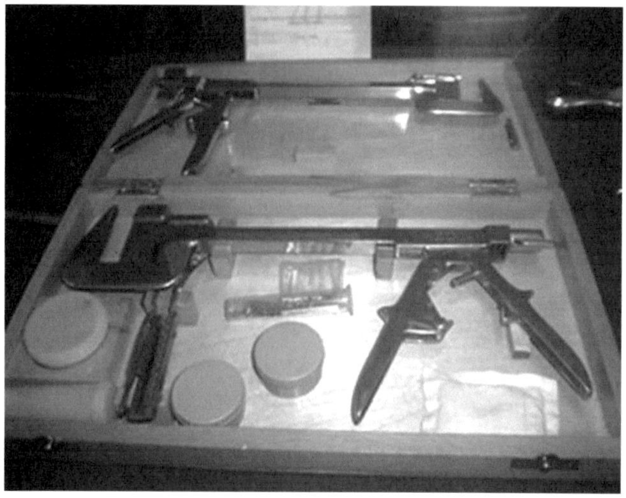

Figure 11. Russian stapler.

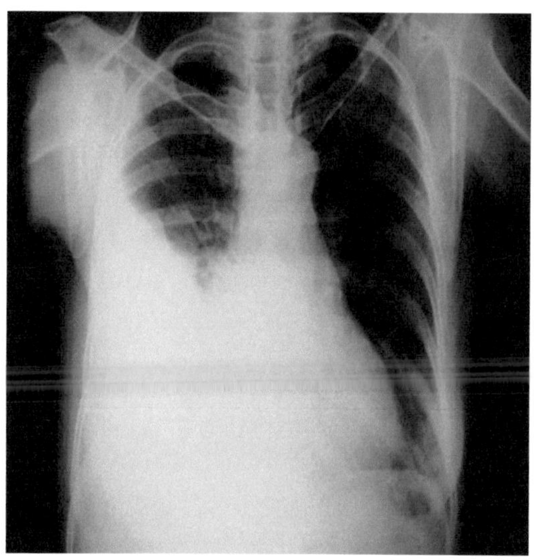

Figure 12. Pleural effusion X-ray image.

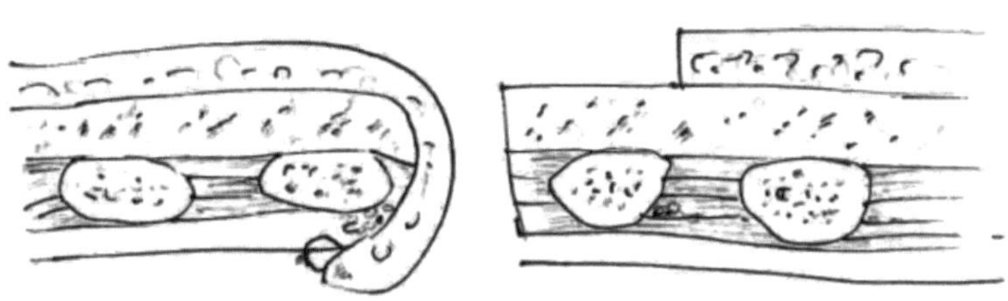

Figure 13. Drainage of the pleural cavity by communicating the pleural cavity to the outside through an incision.

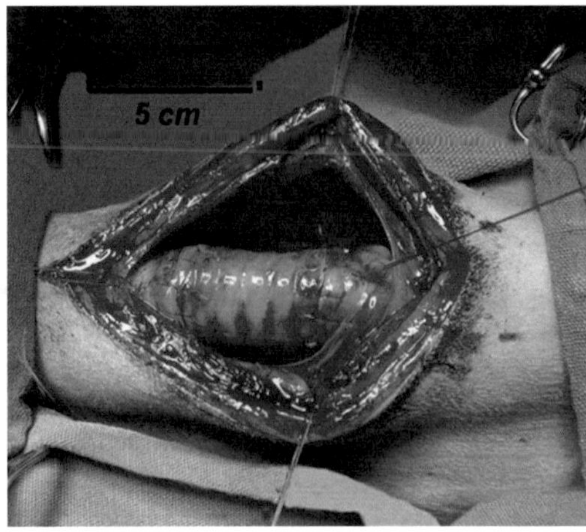

Figure 14. Tracheal surgery.

this section, we must indicate and contraindicate methods such as video-assisted and robotic surgeries.

In addition, although drug administration is not a surgical procedure, the synergy of drugs based on studies of molecular biology for the treatment of chronic-degenerative diseases will be very important.

4. Contraindications of video-thoracoscopic surgery

4.1. Video-assisted surgery/robotic surgery

Currently, there are many surgical subspecialties and technological advances, that is, chest surgery procedures such as pleural decortication, pulmonary resection, endocavitary aspiration, and transbronchial punctures are performed in order to obtain lymph node tissue through video-assisted surgery (**Tables 2** and **3**) [7].

As of today, the long-distance surgery along with robotic surgery will be preponderant in the future. The large number of subspecialties currently underway should be noted, that is, surgical oncology, interventional bronchoscopy, or cochlear implants and surgeons must become subspecialists with genetic and robotic multitraining.

The medicine of the future plus multiple technological changes will force a student who chooses a medical degree to rely on genomics, molecular biology, epigenetics, computer networks and telecommunications, bioelectronics, artificial intelligence, communication and psycho-medical sciences, treatment techniques, geriatrics, preventive medicine, administration, and health economics and ethics. Likewise, the health professional will need to be competent in selecting worthy information from millions of data published daily. It is also

Advantages	Disadvantages
Lesser traumatic interventions	Difficult access in deep lesions
Better postoperative recovery	Increased possibility of leaving hidden disease
Faster functional recovery	More postoperative follow-up due to increased chance of hidden disease
Better immune response	Greater difficulty in the evaluation of surgical margins.
Quicker reincorporation to full activity	
Lower economic cost	

Table 2. Advantages and disadvantages of video-thoracoscopic surgery [7].

Absolute	Relative
Dense pleural symphysis	Significant hilar lymphadenopathy
Absence of pleural space	Mayor emphysema
Inability of achieving ipsilateral pulmonary collapse	Nodular lesions less than 1 cm deep
Inability of tolerating monopulmonary ventilation	Tumor size greater than 5 cm
Decompensated cardiovascular disease	Chest wall involvement
Thrombocytopenia of less than 60,000 or INR greater than 20	Serious deformity of the thoracic cage
Inadequate visualization and instrumentation	Radiotherapy or neoadjuvant chemotherapy

Table 3. Contraindications of video-thoracoscopic surgery [7].

important to point out that the knowledge obtained will be added to information in the basic subjects, and both will enable the medical student to prevent some diseases like diabetes. All this accumulation of knowledge will mean that the medicine of the future will be practiced by groups of specialists and subspecialists, as it is already being done in some countries; conceivably, individual practice is going to decrease significantly.

The book of the General Health Council entitled "Futures of the formation of human resources for health in Mexico" by Dr. Enrique Ruelas Barajas, Dr. Antonio Alonso Concheiro, and Guadalupe Alarcón Fuentes has been fundamental to integrate this topic. It includes references from complementary medicine (herbal and acupuncture), which, in some European countries, is already part of the medical profession. Some groups of professionals even include specialists in administration and health economics [8].

Finally, some sensible words about medical ethics must be mentioned: this discipline derived from philosophy has grown in a very important way and is surely going to increase every day, mainly because of the positive complexity of technological development.

In accordance with Louie et al., which report an early experience with robotic lung resection, it resulted in similar outcomes when compared with mature video-assisted thoracoscopic surgery (VATS) cases. However, a potential benefit of robotics may relate to postoperative pain reduction ($p = 0.039$), and early return to usual activities ($p = 0.001$) was shorter in the robotic group [9].

The Spanish Royal Academy defines a robot as a programmable electronic machine with the capacity to manipulate objects and carry out operations that only the human being is capable of doing. In this regard, it is also known that the word robot derives from the word robota, which in Czechoslovakia designates "compulsive work." These words appeared in the play Rossum's *Universal Robots* written in 1921 by Karem Kapeq, a story about the sudden inability for humans to reproduce and a war between robots and humans [10]. On the other hand, the American Institute of Robotics expresses the following idea of a robot: a machine of human form that performs the tasks of a human being, but without sensitivity. Meanwhile, the University of Nebraska in the United States was one of the earliest institutions to employ distance-assistance methods in the 1950s. It was until 1986 that the first satellite program was launched by the Mayo Clinic in Rochester, Minnesota, and the Scottsdale Clinic in Arizona. These facts gave rise to the era of telemedicine that would later establish the foundation of remote surgery.

The concept of robotic surgery with telepresence was born by the effort and collaboration of the Research Institute of Stanford University, NASA, and the United States Department of Defense to treat wounded soldiers. This technology was initially assigned to the neurosurgeons, and in 1985 the first surgical procedure with a robot was performed with the Mitsubishi system to obtain a brain biopsy through stereotaxy.

In 1988, the PROBOT system was created in England to aid in a transurethral prostatic resection. It consisted of the elaboration of a three-dimensional model of the prostate where the surgeon delineated the limits of the resection and the robot calculated the trajectories of the incisions. In 1992, IBM produced a robot called ROBODOC for orthopedic interventions; the number of surgeries performed by this method increased with hip replacement surgery.

In Mexico City in 1996, two cholecystectomies were operated from a distance of 10 m by a robotic arm with 6° of pronosupination.

In November 2001, a robotic arm was used to assist in a hysterectomy [11].

In 1997, Dr. Garcia Ruiz of Mexico and Dr. Falcone of the Cleveland Clinic performed the first remote robotic surgery that consisted of a tubal reanastomosis. This performance demonstrated the feasibility of making endoscopic sutures, which surgeons said were faster and more accurate. In 1996, at the Mexican Institute of Social Security of Tijuana, doctors Carvajal and Fogel performed a laparoscopic cholecystectomy in porcine models.

In 2001, the Zeus project (a system of robotic instruments) performed hiatus and gall-bladder operations [12].

Unfortunately, the cost of a robot, which is around one million dollars, increases the costs of surgeries. For example, the costs of the Da Vinci system are higher than of a laparoscopy, and some doctors refer to the robot as "expensive toy."

Hopefully, robot systems will be smaller in the future and, therefore, cheaper.

Swanson et al. [13] compared hospital cost and clinical outcomes for lobectomies by video-assisted thoracic surgery (VATS) and wedge resections versus robot-assisted (RATS) lobectomies. Data from 15,502 surgeries were analyzed. The average cost of inpatient procedures with RATS was $25,040.70 US Dls versus $20476.60 for VATS ($p = 0.0001$) for lobectomies and $19,592.40 versus $16,600.10 ($p = 0.0001$) for wedge resections. Inpatient operating times were longer for RATS lobectomy than for VATS lobectomy (4.49 vs. 4.23 h; $p = 0.959$) and wedge resection (3.26 vs. 2.86 h; $p = 0.003$). The length of stay was similar with no differences in adverse events. They concluded that RATS lobectomy and wedge resection seem to have higher hospital cost and longer operating times, without any differences in adverse events.

Resection with robot seems to be an appropriate alternative for VATS and with better results than with an open surgery [14].

> *"Robotic lobectomy for cancer offers excellent results, with excellent lymph node removal with minimal morbidity, mortality and pain. Despite its costs, it is cost-effective for the hospital system. Disadvantages include capital costs, equipment learning curve, and lack of lung palpation. Robotic surgery is an important tool in the arsenal for the thoracic surgeon, but its precise function continues to evolve" [15].*

General thorax surgery was a series of maneuvers especially indicated in pulmonary tuberculosis, so it is not possible to describe a technique without describing the pathology indicated. This treatment was carried out, as has been mentioned before, in the past, because today the drug treatment is very useful in tuberculosis.

Currently, lung cancer, which is the main cause of hospitalization and the invasive methods that apply to this disease, has advanced very importantly as video-assisted surgery and surgery performed with a robot.

Histopathological diagnoses vary in lung cancer. These techniques are being applied for diagnosis, and therefore the treatment is modified. Immunohistochemical techniques help improve and personalize the patient's treatment. For these histological studies, a sample can be taken by video-assisted surgery, and in some pulmonary resections surgery with a robot is practiced. Biopsies taken by VATS are possible in the topographic areas of the thorax, and with robotic surgery it is possible to perform pulmonary excision and, if necessary, pneumonectomy. There is no doubt that with VATS and RATS (robotic surgery), the advance has been of great importance because the incisions are small, and the days of hospital stay also and the costs in the VATS have decreased, but unfortunately this has not been so in the RATS. Undoubtedly, this type of treatment in general chest surgery will change radically because of the important advance that the technology has had. It is currently possible to detect pathology that in previous years was not feasible to diagnose. The latest publications on these topics of surgery describe them favorably and the results on VATS and RATS also; new generations of human resources must be very attentive to technological changes and should be mentally prepared to learn and perform this type of surgery. However, a very important doctors′ complaint is the impossibility of palpating some of the pathologies. There is no doubt that this situation will be solved "with a new technology" that tells us the organs′ consistency or about hidden ganglia.

According to different opinions from 2020 to 2030, there will be several disciplines that currently do not exist in the curriculum of students due to scientific and technological advances [8].

As I mentioned in the previous lines, surgery and armed interventions have been practiced more in pulmonary tuberculosis in the past and currently in lung cancer and chronic-degenerative conditions.

There is no doubt that knowledge, technology, and the spirit of research have achieved this progress in addition to the progress in basic matters such as molecular biology, epigenetics, immunology, and so on. In brief, there will be further great progress. Many physical examinations can be achieved in lung cancer patients using the mediastinoscope and fibrobronchoscopes. Fortunately, different types of antibodies that are tested for diagnostic purpose have been found and will, surely, have very positive effects.

An example I find very illustrating can be found on page 241 of the book "The Shock of the Future" by Alvin Toffler. The biochemist Marvin Johnson from the University of Wisconsin wrote: "Recently, microorganisms have been domesticated because human did not know its existence" [16]. Currently, human not just knows them but gets many benefits from them, that is, large-scale production of vitamins, enzymes, antibiotics, citric acid, and other useful compounds. In a few years, biologists will create microorganisms to feed animals and ultimately humans.

Acknowledgements

The authors are grateful to Miss María de Lourdes Espinosa Cruz for her invaluable dedication and secretarial assistance as well as to Mr. Manuel Silva Alvarado for the elaboration of the drawings.

Author details

Jaime Villalba Caloca[1]*, Avelina Sotres Vega[1], Javier Pineda Gutiérrez[1], Sergio Martínez Fonseca[1], Marcelino Alonso Gómez[1] and Bettina Sommer Cervantes[2]

*Address all correspondence to: jaimevc@iner.gob.mx

1 Experimental Lung Transplantation Research Unit, National Institute of Respiratory Diseases, Mexico City, Mexico

2 Department of Bronchial Hyperreactivity, National Institute of Respiratory Diseases, Mexico City, Mexico

References

[1] Villalba-Caloca J. Cirugía de tórax en México. Neumologia y Cirugía de Tórax. 2010;**69**: 46-53

[2] Cárdenas de la Peña E, editor. Del sanatorio de Huipulco, al Instituto Nacional de Enfermedades Respiratorias cincuenta años. Unique edition. México: INER; 1986. 328 p

[3] Salazar-Lezama MA, Valdez-Vázquez R, Villareal-Velarde H, Torres-Cruz A, López-Segundo E. In: Cano-Valle F, Ibarra-Pérez C, Morales-Gómez J, editors. Tuberculósis pulmonar. 1st ed. España: Elsiever; 2006. pp. 103-114

[4] Jiménez M. Nociones de fisiología. Unique ed. Stylo: México; 1954. 673 p

[5] Monaldi V. Lotta contro la Tuberculosi. 9: No. 9 (Sept), 1938

[6] Vara-Cuadrado F. Apuntes históricos sobre la cirugía de la tuberculosis pulmonar en el siglo XX. Revista de Patología Respiratoria. 2005;**8**:3-16

[7] Gutiérrez E, Ortíz CA, Gómez J, Duitama J, DíazJ J, Fernández MR, Field RA, García F, García CC. Situación actual de la cirugía videoasistida. Revista Colombiana de Cirugía. 2013;**28**:212-222

[8] Ruelas-Barajas E, Concheiro-Alonso A, Fuentes-Alarcón G, editors. Futuros de la formación de recursos humanos para la salud en México 2005-2050. Consejo de Salubridad General. 1st ed. México: Láser SA de CV; 2005. 85 p

[9] Louie B, Farivar A, Aye R, Valliéres E. Early experience with robotic lung resection results in similar operative outcomes and morbidity when compared with matched video-assisted thoracoscopic surgery cases. The Annals of Thoracic Surgery. 2012;**93**:1598-1605. DOI: 10.1016/j.athoracsur.2012.01.067

[10] Zjawinskisonia Zjawinski S. Rossum's universal robots is revived in New York, culture. 07.05.0701:16 pm. https://www.wired.com/2007/07/rossums-univers/

[11] Dueñas-García OF, Rico-Olvera H, Beltrán-Montoya JJ. Telemedicina y cirugía robótica. Ginecología y Obstetricia de México. 2008;**76**:161-166

[12] Carbajal-Ramos A. Cirugía Robótica. Cirujano General. 2003;**25**:311-320

[13] Swanson S, Miller D, McKenna RJ, Howington J, Marshall BM, Yoo CA, Moore M, Gunnarsson CL, Meyers BF. Comparing robot-assisted thoracic surgical lobectomy with conventional video-assisted thoracic lobectomy and wedge resection: Results from a multihospital database (premier). The Journal of Thoracic and Cardiovascular Surgery. 2014;**147**:929-937

[14] Basil S, Bryant A, Minnich D, Wei B, Cerfolio R. Performing robotic lobectomy and segmentectomy: Cost, profitability and outcomes. The Annals of Thoracic Surgery. 2014; **98**:203-209. DOI: 10.1016/j.athoracsur.2014.02.051

[15] Kent M, Wang T, Whyte R, Curran T, Flores R, Gangadharan S. Open, video-assisted thoracic surgery and robotic lobectomy: Review of a national database. The Annals of Thoracic Surgery. 2014;**97**:236-244. DOI: 10.1016/j.athoracsur.2013.07117

[16] Toffler A. El schok del futuro, 10th ed. España: Plaza Janes SA; 1979. 241 p